T0210875

SpringerBriefs in Computer Science

More information about this series at http://www.springer.com/series/10028

Feng Xia · Azizur Rahim

MAC Protocols
for Cyber-Physical Systems

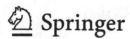
Springer

Feng Xia
Dalian University of Technology
Dalian
China

Azizur Rahim
Dalian University of Technology
Dalian
China

ISSN 2191-5768   ISSN 2191-5776   (electronic)
SpringerBriefs in Computer Science
ISBN 978-3-662-46360-4   ISBN 978-3-662-46361-1   (eBook)
DOI 10.1007/978-3-662-46361-1

Library of Congress Control Number: 2015940979

Springer Heidelberg New York Dordrecht London

Printed on acid-free paper

Springer-Verlag GmbH Berlin Heidelberg is part of Springer Science+Business Media
(www.springer.com)

Preface

Cyber-Physical Systems (CPS) is one of the most promising directions in the field of information and communication technologies. It has attracted intensive attention and participation from both industry and from academia in the past few years. CPS are integrations of computation, networking, and physical dynamics, in which embedded devices are networked to sense, monitor, and control the physical world. This radical transformation from stand-alone devices to networked systems facilitates various innovative applications, not only on a large scale but also for personal and micro-level use. To fully explore the potential of CPS, however, various applications including Wireless Body Area Networks (WBANs) require high Quality of Services (QoS) in terms of timeliness, reliability, energy efficiency, and other metrics. Medium Access Control (MAC) layer plays a critical role in meeting these requirements. For instance, reliability can be achieved with enhanced scheduling schemes, appropriate channel access protocols, improved schemes for retransmission, and optimal packet size at MAC layer. The major objective of this book is to examine the challenges and issues at MAC layer with an in-depth analysis of state-of-the-art protocols based on IEEE 802.15.4. In addition, this book also presents the design and evaluation of an adaptive MAC protocol for medical CPS, which exemplifies how to achieve real-time and reliable communications in CPS by exploiting IEEE 802.15.4-based MAC protocols. This book will be of interest to researchers, practitioners, and students to better understand the QoS requirements of CPS at MAC sublayer.

Over the years there have been many people working in the field of CPS. The literature helped us gain the knowledge necessary for our research, which makes this book possible. We would like to thank Xiangjie Kong, Tie Qiu, Ruixia Gao, Linqiang Wang, Ruonan Hao, Yang Cao, Lei Xue, Daqiang Zhang, Daojing He, Alexey Vinel, Nadeem Javaid, Muhammad Aslam, Ziaur Rahman, U. Qasim, and Z.A. Khan for their contributions to the work reported in this book. We are grateful to all members of the Mobile and Social Computing Laboratory, as well as to Asim

Idrees and Muhammad Farshad Panhwar for their help in realizing this book. This work is partially supported by Natural Science Foundation of China under Grant No. 60903153.

Dalian, China   Feng Xia
September 2014   Azizur Rahim

Contents

Acronyms

ABE	Adaptive Backoff Exponent
ACK	Acknowledgment
AGBA	Adaptive Guard Band Algorithm
BAN	Body Area Network
BE	Backoff Exponent
BER	Bit Error Rate
BI	Beacon Interval
BO	Beacon Order
CAP	Contention Access Period
CCA	Clear Channel Assessment
CCAP	Configurable Contention Access Period
CDMA	Code Division Multiple Access
CE	Consumer Electronics
CFP	Contention Free Period
CPS	Cyber-Physical Systems
CSMA	Carries Sense Multiple Access
CSMA/CA	Carries Sense Multiple Access with Collision Avoidance
CTS	Clear To Send
CW	Contention Window
DAF	Drift Adjustment Factor
ECG	ElectroCardioGram
EDF	Earliest Deadline First
EEG	ElectroEncephaloGram
FDMA	Frequency Division Multiple Access
FFD	Full Function Device
FRT	Frame Tailoring
GTS	Guaranteed Time Slots
IFS	InterFrame Spacing
ISM	Industrial, Scientific, and Medical
LIFS	Long InterFrame Space
LPL	Low Power Listening

MAC	Medium Access Control
MCPS	Medical Cyber-Physical Systems
MICS	Medical Implant Communication Service
MN	Master Node
MPDU	MAC Protocol Data Unit
MS	Monitoring Station
MSDU	MAC Service Data Unit
NB	Backoff Number
NC	Network Control
OSI	Open Systems Interconnection
PAN	Personal Area Network
PHY	Physical
QoS	Quality of Service
RF	Radio Frequency
RFD	Reduce Function Device
RPD	Remaining Permissable Delay
RTS	Ready To Send
SD	Superframe Duration
SIFS	Short Interframe Space
SO	Superframe Order
TDMA	Time Division Multiple Access
TSRB	Time Slot Reserved for Burst traffic
TSRP	Time Slot Reserved for Periodic traffic
TTP	Time Triggered Protocol
UWB	Ultra-Wide Band
WBAN	Wireless Body Area Network
WMTS	Wireless Medical Telemetry Services
WSAN	Wireless Sensor and Actuator Network
WSN	Wireless Sensor Network

Chapter 1
Introduction

Abstract We are currently on the brink of a revolutionary transformation from stand-alone, self-contained embedded systems to Cyber-Physical Systems (CPS), an exciting new domain after the Internet. In CPS, numerous embedded devices with limited computational, communication, sensing capacities, and power supply are networked, enabling a variety of innovative applications that were even unimaginable several years ago. This chapter presents a brief introduction to CPS, its applications, and requirements. Taking wireless body area network (WBAN) as an illustrative case of CPS (for healthcare), we discuss system architecture, design requirements, and energy consumption in the context of WBAN. In order to achieve high efficiency, a number of protocols and solutions have been proposed so far; however, efforts are still needed to overcome the challenges and requirements. In addition to the major requirements of WBANs such as reliability and scalability, these proposed solutions should be able to tackle energy dissipation caused by different sources of energy wastage.

Keywords Cyber-physical systems · Healthcare · Embedded systems · Sensors

1.1 Cyber-Physical Systems

The revolutionary developmental growth from stand-alone embedded systems to networked systems has led to new trends in the field of information and communication technologies. One of the most promising directions, which bridges real world's physical objects and virtual cyber world's computation and communication processes, is CPS, where networked embedded devices control the physical objects with feedback from physical objects to computation and vice versa [1]. For example, in industrial applications, a number of sensor nodes are attached to machines to communicate machines' status to a computation core which sends the feedback control/command to actuators attached to machines. This radical transformation from stand-alone devices to (generally large-scale) networked systems yields considerable challenges, including, for example, resource constraints, dynamic network topology, platform heterogeneity, and mixed traffic [2].

© The Author(s) 2015   1
F. Xia and A. Rahim, *MAC Protocols for Cyber-Physical Systems*,
SpringerBriefs in Computer Science, DOI 10.1007/978-3-662-46361-1_1

1.1.1 What Is CPS?

The world we are living in has seen mutations of many typical mechanical systems to computer-controlled and networked complex electromechanical systems. The rapid growth in networking, processing, storage, and control capabilities has given rise to the emergence of highly collaborative CPS. Some defining characteristics of CPS [3–6] include cyber capability in physical components, networking at multiple and extreme scales, complexity at multiple temporal and spatial scales, dynamic reorganization and reconfiguration, high degrees of automation, closed control loops at multiple scales, unconventional computational and physical substrates, and dependable even certifiable operations. These kinds of human artifacts enable ubiquitous networking and connectivity to control mechanical systems using embedded processors. The environmental states are sensed and controlled using sensors and actuators for a diverse range of applications [6]. CPS provide interaction to physical world which must be safe, secure, efficient, and dependable. This intimate coupling of cyber and physical worlds can vary in both scale and size, for, e.g., smartphones to smart industrial applications.

As shown in Fig. 1.1, the physical world's processes and the cyber computation world are bridged with feedback loops, where the computation processes affect physical processes, and vice versa. As we know that the physical world is not entirely predictable, close interaction of the cyber world is required to control and monitor physical processes and objects efficiently. The coordination of physical resources and cyber world yields remarkable capabilities from personal to society-scale applications. Meanwhile, this radical transformation and integration is accompanied by considerable challenges and requirements.

A typical CPS consists of the following components: physical objects/applications, actuators, sensors, communication, and computing core. These graphically deployed sensors and actuators are bridged with communication and computing core. The state information are collected and sent to computing core via communication networks, possibly a combination of multiple networks including, e.g., wireless sensor networks (WSNs) or wireless sensor and actuator networks (WSANs). These communication networks enable the reliable and real-time communication of data. The computing core is responsible for decision making to generate control commands based on the collected information. The computing core may be centralized or

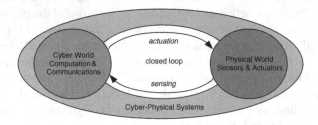

Fig. 1.1 Coupling of physical and cyber worlds

distributed to facilitate the operation of CPS. The control commands are sent using the communication networks to proper actuators. In this manner, the combination of these sensors/actuators, communication networks, and computing core enables to bridge the cyber world with physical systems/applications.

1.1.2 Applications

Traditionally, embedded systems have been used to integrate physical processes with computing [7, 8]. Such kind of embedded systems include home appliances, games, automotive electronics, weapons, communication systems, among many others. However, these embedded systems have the deficiency of interaction to outside world and act like "Closed Boxes." The rapid growth of computational capabilities has enabled the radical transformation of these stand-alone systems to network-controlled systems, which we envision.

CPS are engineered systems with physical world interaction, where operations are coordinated, integrated, and controlled by a communication and computing core. This coupling provides solutions for different applications, not only on large scale but also for personal use and at microlevel. Like transformation of human interaction via Internet, CPS will enable the physical world to interact with the cyber world, thus transforming how human beings interact with the physical world [8]. Applications of CPS include, e.g., medical healthcare, home automation, environmental control, assisted living, smart city, transportation, traffic control, process control, automotive systems, defense systems, water supply, smart grid, robotics, smart spaces, energy conservation, smart factory, industrial automation, battlefield surveillance, communication systems, and aerospace systems, to mention a few.

With increasing demands for ubiquitous and high-quality healthcare services, for instance, medical CPS over Wireless Body Area Networks (WBANs) has emerged as a promising solution for advanced healthcare services. Medical CPS is an integration of the sensing, communication, computing, and medical processes. Besides conventional embedded systems, equipment networking, and health monitoring systems, medical CPS offers a multitude of opportunities for WBANs to facilitate ubiquitous and mobile healthcare. Section 1.2 presents WBANs as a case of CPS to visualize the applications of CPS.

1.1.3 General Requirements

Reliability and efficiency have been of great interest for humans in the modern era. The use of embedded systems and computer-controlled applications has greatly improved reliability and efficiency. However, radical transformation of stand-alone devices to network-controlled devices has lead to higher expectation for improved reliability and efficiency in the context of CPS. For deployment of CPS in real-time applications, e.g., healthcare and monitoring, reliability and efficiency should be of great concern while developing protocols and standards; otherwise, deployment of CPS for such applications will not be convincing.

To achieve the specific QoS (Quality of Service) requirements for different applications, the performance depends upon the underlying network infrastructure. For example, in healthcare systems, the information from human body should be transferred to the coordinator and then health services provider for timely precautionary measurement and prescription. However, if raise of glucose level in blood is not timely reported and the insulin actuator is not activated on time to inject the required insulin to control the blood sugar level, the patient's health might be harmed, which is not acceptable for today's highly demanding healthcare systems [9]. Similarly, packet loss and information delay in such applications may not be acceptable sometimes. In contrast, in temperature monitoring systems, like the one used to control room temperature, this may be acceptable.

As the real-world objects and applications are not entirely predictable, the emerging CPS should not be operating in a fixed manner. It must have the ability to cope with the unexpected conditions. Adaptability and robustness should be considered before deployment of CPS to real-time applications. In order to accommodate newly added subsystem or modification, CPS also require scalability, not only on small scale but also for complex applications like smart factory where progressive work takes place with the passage of time.

In order to achieve the highest level of satisfaction for applications' requirements, metrics like timeliness, robustness, security, reliability, predictability, efficiency, and many others can be used to define QoS. The level of satisfaction varies for different applications depending upon the natural and environmental factors. In general, delay, jitter, throughput, and packet loss are the most fundamental characteristics to define the degree of satisfaction in cyber world [10–14].

1.2 Wireless Body Area Networks: A Case of CPS

To achieve efficient and effective healthcare services within hospitals or outside, CPS facilitate to bridge on-body, in-body, or around the human body sensor nodes and computing cores for ubiquitous and mobile healthcare. Advancement in storage and wireless technologies has facilitated the production of small devices with long-term capabilities of sensing and monitoring. CPS built upon WBAN is a networking concept that enables us to use these portable, small, and lightweight sensor nodes to monitor physiological signals for a long period of time. These energy-constrained small devices are used to measure the human body's physiological signs. These measurements are communicated using the communication capabilities for prescription or diagnosis of these physiological signs by a medical practitioner. Energy consumption is one of the most important factors to be considered for data streaming to the monitoring station via wireless communication channel. Lifespan of these tiny

devices can be prolonged with energy-efficient mechanisms for communication and
signal processing [15].

To measure the physiological signs from human body, tiny sensor nodes are
implanted or attached to the human body. These devices have limited computational
and communication capabilities and power supply. Electroencephalography (EEG),
electrocardiogram (ECG), heartbeat, respiratory patterns, posture, temperature, and
breathing rate are some of the physiological signs to be measured. For data communication of these signs, data rates vary from 1 Kbps to 1 Mbps [16]. The collected
information from human bodies are communicated to an external monitoring station
via in/on or around human's body central controlling device called coordinator. The
architecture of WBAN will be discussed in the following subsection.

Communication of nodes in WBAN can be divided into three categories: communication of on-body node to a remote coordinator, communication between two
on-body sensor nodes, and communication of implanted (in-body) node to on-body
node [17]. These three communication patterns are named off-body, on-body, and
in-body communication, respectively. WBAN can be used for many applications,
including healthcare monitoring, personal entertainment, and worker health condition monitoring for safety.

1.2.1 Architecture

WBANs can be utilized for both medical and non-medical applications. As shown in
Fig. 1.2, communication architecture of WBAN is usually composed of three levels
of communication. Level 1, which is the core level, consists of small sensor nodes
attached or implanted to a human body for long-time monitoring of physiological,
biomedical signs, or human body postures. For medical applications, where physiological signs like EEG, ECG, heartbeat, blood sugar, human body's temperature,
and Blood Pressure (BP) are to be monitored, biosensors will be used. To measure
acceleration and human body mobility, biokinetic sensors can be used. These on, in,
or around human body sensor nodes are organized in most common star topology

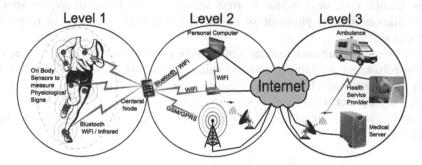

Fig. 1.2 Architecture of WBANs

for communication of sensed information to a central device. The central device communicates the received information for diagnose and prescription from health services provider. For communication, the central node uses existing technologies of Level 1 and Level 2 as shown in Fig. 1.2. Communication pattern in Level 1 is termed as IntraBAN, while communication in Level 2 and Level 3 are termed as ExtraBAN communication.

The number and nature of sensor nodes vary according to application requirements. In deployment of these nodes, human body structure and mobility are kept in consideration for reliable communication. Human body tissues are sensitive to electromagnetic radiation of transceiver. To avoid harmful effects, transceiver's power is adjusted to the minimum possible level. The sensor nodes which are placed on the head and torso do not observe mobility as compared to the nodes placed on head and legs. Sensor nodes attached to legs and arms scrutinize high mobility.

For data communication in Level 1, WBANs use Industrial, Scientific and Medical (ISM) frequency band, Ultra-WideBand (UWB), and Wireless Medical Telemetry Services (WMTS) frequency band. In wideband UWB, because of difficulties in channel access mechanism it is difficult to use Clear Channel Assessment (CCA). Narrow pulses are used to transmit data [14]. Medical Implant Communication Service (MICS) (402–405 MHz) and WMTS (14 MHz) are licensed frequency bands [18]. ISM (2.4 MHz) is an unlicensed frequency band. WMTS is a highly secure spectrum used only by authorized and trained physicians/technicians. WMTS cannot support audio and video streaming. MICS is especially dedicated to implant communication. The most common frequency band used in WBANs is ISM. WiFi, Bluetooth, and ZigBee also use this specific frequency band for wireless communication.

Medical applications and consumer electronics applications depend heavily upon protocol design at Level 1. Small battery-operated sensor nodes collect critical and noncritical information from environment or human body. The traffic flows among these nodes can be classified into: normal traffic, emergency traffic, and on-demand traffic. Normal traffic is generated periodically under normal conditions. Coordinator or central node collects normal traffic periodically. On-body or implanted sensor nodes initiate emergency traffic whenever the measured value exceeds a predefined threshold value. Emergency traffic is unpredictable, and is not generated on regular basis. Central node or coordinator originates on-demand traffic to acquire some information needed by physician or monitoring station for treatment or network management.

The overall performance indicators of WBAN, especially energy efficiency, reliability, robustness, wearability, and scalability, are closely related to Level 1. For energy efficiency and reliability of communication, design of Medium Access Layer (MAC) layer protocols at Level 1 plays a vital role. With an efficient MAC design at Level 1, high throughput, high energy efficiency, and minimum delay can be achieved.

1.2.2 Design Issues

Using the capabilities of in/on or around human body's sensor nodes, noncritical and critical information from different parts of the human body are collected and communicated to the coordinator. To achieve effective health monitoring systems, transmission reliability and latency are very important issues to be considered. Similarly, scalability and energy efficiency are also required to prolong the lifespan of WBAN.

The first goal to be achieved in WBANs is energy efficiency. As the sensor nodes are battery operated with limited computational and communication capabilities, energy dissipation at Level 1 should be reduced as much as possible to achieve uninterrupted long-time patient monitoring. To prolong the lifespan of these tiny sensor nodes, adaptive and dynamic mechanisms should be used with efficient utilization of resources.

Power consumption of sensor node's transceiver is one of the dominant sources to be considered in WBANs. Power consumption of transceiver can be reduced with proper optimization of physical (PHY) and MAC layer processes. Power optimization at PHY layer often has some limitations. Proper approaches at MAC layer like enhanced channel access techniques, optimal packet structure, smart signaling techniques, and multiple transmission scheduling schemes may result in improved power efficiency.

Packet loss probability and transmission delay of packets contribute to reliability of WBANs. Packet loss probability depends upon Bit Error Rate (BER) of the channel and packet transmission procedures at MAC layer. Reliability of WBANs can be achieved with enhanced scheduling schemes, appropriate channel access protocols, improved schemes for retransmission and optimal packet size at MAC layer. In addition, MAC layer has the capability to achieve scalability in WBANs. Without proper support for scalability at MAC layer, increasing or decreasing the number of sensor nodes in WBANs may result in degraded network performance in terms of packet loss and delay, which is not acceptable for monitoring of life-critical physiological signs.

Different applications of health monitoring systems require different QoS. To achieve high QoS for various applications, MAC layer plays a vital role. For instance, deterministic packet loss and packet delay can be achieved using Time division multiple access (TDMA) and polling channel access mechanisms at MAC layer. Carrier-sense multiple access with collision avoidance (CSMA/CA) can be utilized at MAC layer for dynamic allocation of transmission channel to end nodes. In contention-based protocols like carrier-sense multiple access (CSMA), adaptive sleep cycles can enhance energy efficiency at the cost of increased packet drop and latency.

1.2.3 Energy Dissipation

As mentioned above, power consumption of sensor nodes in WBANs is one of the main issues to be addressed efficiently. Deployed sensor nodes often have limited power resources, and in most cases it is not possible to recharge or to replace them. The power dissipation due to overhearing of nodes, idle listening, packet collision, protocol overhead, state switching of the transceiver, and packet forwarding can be reduced by introducing low power protocols at MAC layer.

Simultaneous transmission of packets from two sensor nodes over a single communication channel results in packets collision at the receiver end. Packets are hence dropped by the receiver and retransmitted by the sender nodes. This retransmission of data/control packets leads to extra energy dissipation. Overhearing is the second source of energy dissipation in WBANs, where the sensor nodes receive data packets for which they are not supposed to receive. These received packets are of no interest for the receiving nodes and are dropped, resulting in extra energy consumption. A third source of energy dissipation is idle listening, where nodes listen to idle communication channel for possible data/control packets to be received. Control packet overhead not only results in extra power consumption but also results in decreased effective throughput of the network. Packet forwarding is considered as a source of energy dissipation in WSN. Nevertheless, due to single-hop communication in star topology in WBANs, it may be ignored. The last but not the least source of energy dissipation is state switching, which occurs when the sensor node's transceiver is switched off/on to avoid idle listening and overhearing. Energy dissipation is increased with frequent switching of transceiver. In order to overcome these sources of energy dissipation and maximize the energy efficiency of WBANs, MAC protocols with efficient scheduling and transmission mechanism need to be designed.

1.3 Overview of the Book

In this Chapter, we first introduce CPS and discuss its applications and general requirements. Rather than jumping directly to the MAC layer, first we introduce WBAN, one of the most important applications of CPS, with focus on its architecture, design issues, and challenges. Chapter 2 provides the classification of MAC protocols, followed by an introduction to some representative protocols (which are not based on IEEE 802.15.4) for WBANs. The performance of IEEE 802.15.4 MAC protocol in the context of CPS is evaluated in Chap. 3. For this purpose, the network QoS is characterized by several metrics, including effective data rate, packet loss rate, and end-to-end delay. These metrics are examined with respect to different MAC parameter settings. A lot of efforts have been made in the literature to overcome the limitations of IEEE 802.15.4. In Chap. 4, an overview of some interesting mechanisms used in existing adaptive and real-time protocols built upon IEEE

802.15.4 is presented. Based on the observations gained from the previous chapters, in Chap. 5, we present an adaptive MAC protocol for medical CPS built on top of IEEE 802.15.4 to achieve reliable and real-time communication. Finally, we present the book summary with open issues in Chap. 6.

References

1. Wolf W (2009) Cyber-physical systems. IEEE Comput. doi:10.1109/MC.2009.81
2. Xia F, Ma L, Dong J, Sun Y (2008) Network QoS management in cyber-physical systems. In: International conference on embedded software and systems symposia. doi:10.1109/ICESS. Symposia.84
3. Poovendran R (2010) Cyber-physical systems: close encounters between two parallel worlds. Proc IEEE. doi:10.1109/JPROC.2010.2050377
4. Rajkumar R, Lee I, Sha L, Stankovic J (2010) Cyber-physical systems: the next computing evolution. In: Proceedings of the 47th design automation conference. ACM, New York
5. Kang KD, Son SH (2008) Real-time data services for cyber physical systems. In: 28th international conference on distributed computing systems workshops. doi:10.1109/ICDCS. Workshops.2008.21
6. Ordinez L, Alimenti O, Rinland E, Gomez M, Marchetti J (2013) Modeling and specifying requirements for cyber-physical systems. IEEE Lat Am Trans 11(1):625–632. doi:10.1109/ TLA.2013.6502874
7. Kim KD, Kumar PR (2012) Cyber-physical systems: a perspective at the centennial. Proc IEEE. doi:10.1109/JPROC.2012.2189792
8. Sztipanovits J (2011) Model integration and cyber physical systems: a semantics perspective. Formal methods, Springer. doi:10.1007/978-3-642-21437-0_1
9. Xia F, Zhao W, Sun Y, Tian YC (2007) Fuzzy logic control based QoS management in wireless sensor/actuator networks. Sensors 7(12):3179–3191. doi:10.1109/ISORC.2011.2160929
10. Lee EA (2008) Cyber physical systems: design challenges. In: 11th IEEE international symposium on object oriented real-time distributed computing (ISORC). doi:10.1109/ISORC.2008. 25
11. Derler P, Lee EA, Vincentelli AS (2012) Modeling cyber-physical systems. Proc IEEE. doi:10. 1109/JPROC.2011.2160929
12. Sha L, Gopalakrishnan S, Liu X, Wang Q (2009) Cyber-physical systems: a new frontier., Machine learning in cyber trustSpringer, New York. doi:10.1007/978-0-387-88735-7_1
13. Shi J, Wan J, Yan H, Suo H (2011) Survey of cyber-physical systems. In: International conference on wireless communications and signal processing (WCSP). doi:10.1109/WCSP.2011. 6096958
14. Mahapatro J, Misra S, Mahadevappa M, Islam N (2014) Interference-aware MAC scheduling and admission control for multiple mobile WBANs used in healthcare monitoring. Int J Commun Syst 28(7):1352–1366. doi:10.1002/dac.2768
15. Alam MM, Berder O, Menard D, Sentieys O (2012) Latency-energy optimized MAC protocol for body sensor networks. In: Ninth international conference on wearable and implantable body sensor networks (BSN). doi:10.1109/BSN.2012.8
16. Ullah S, Higgins H, Braem B, Latre B, Blondia C, Moerman I, Saleem S, Rahman Z, Kwak KS (2012) Comprehensive survey of wireless body area networks. J Med Syst 36(3):1065–1094. doi:10.1007/s10916-010-9571-3
17. Thotahewa KMS, Redoute JM, Yuce MR (2014) Ultra wideband wireless body area networks. Springer, New York. ISBN: 978-3-319-05286-1
18. Islam MN, Khan J, Yuce MR (2013) A MAC protocol for implanted devices communication in the MICS band. In: IEEE international conference on body sensor networks (BSN). doi:10. 1109/BSN.2013.6575463

Chapter 2
MAC Protocols

Abstract Resource efficiency is one of the most important factors that should be considered when developing a MAC protocol for CPS like WBAN. This chapter presents the critical literature review of different approaches used to design MAC protocols to minimize energy consumption. Control packet overhead of communication, idle listening of nodes to receive expected data packets, overhearing, and collision of data packets are the major sources of energy dissipation in WBANs. A versatile MAC protocol should have the capabilities to minimize energy dissipation in aforementioned situations. An introduction of typical MAC protocols (which are not based on IEEE 802.15.4) for WBAN is presented in this chapter with focus on their strengths and weaknesses.

Keywords Medium access · Multiple access · Communication overhead · Overhearing · Contention

2.1 Introduction

MAC is a sublayer of data link layer commonly known as layer 2 of Open Systems Interconnection (OSI) model. MAC sublayer is responsible for a number of functions including addressing and channel access controlling mechanism. For multiple nodes in a network to communicate through shared medium, MAC sublayer provides channel access control mechanism known as multiple access protocol. For short-range wireless communications in CPS (e.g., WSN, WSAN, and WBAN), MAC protocols often use Time Division Multiple Access (TDMA) or Carries Sense Multiple Access with Collision Avoidance (CSMA/CA) for fair access of shared medium. Frequency Division Multiple Access (FDMA) and Code Division Multiple Access (CDMA) are not supposed to be suitable mechanisms to access the shared medium in CPS like WBAN due to hardware complexity and high power consumption. In case WBANs are not dynamic by nature, CSMA/CA will not be a suitable choice. On the other hand, TDMA-based approaches consume extra energy for synchronization. Design of MAC protocols varies according to the applications' requirements. This chapter, which is based on our paper published in the seventh International

© The Author(s) 2015   11
F. Xia and A. Rahim, *MAC Protocols for Cyber-Physical Systems*,
SpringerBriefs in Computer Science, DOI 10.1007/978-3-662-46361-1_2

Table 2.1 CSMA/CA and TDMA comparison

Feature	CSMA/CA	TDMA
Power consumption	High	Low
Traffic level support	Low	High
Bandwidth utilization	Low	Maximum
Synchronization	N/A	Necessary
Mobility (Dynamic)	Good	Poor

Conference on Broadband, Wireless Computing, Communication and Applications (BWCCA 2012) [1], provides in-depth analysis of different existing approaches used to design MAC protocols that are not based on IEEE 802.15.4. MAC protocols that explore IEEE 802.15.4 will be covered in the following chapters. Table 2.1 presents the comparison of CSMA/CA and TDMA approaches.

It is worth noting that IEEE 802.15.4a is a low data rate standard which defines PHY and MAC layer specifications [2]. This standard is adopted for many applications [3, 4]. Another related standard is IEEE 802.15.6 [5], which defines the PHY and MAC layer specification to be used for in-body or on-body sensor nodes communication via UWB. This standard operates in three modes: beacon-enabled mode with superframe boundaries, nonbeacon-enabled with superframe boundaries, and nonbeacon-enabled without superframe boundaries. Due to the required complex and power demanding transceiver at sensor node, this standard does not suit WBANs investigated in this book.

2.2 Classification of MAC Protocols

MAC protocols for CPS like WBAN can be categorized into three categories based on the underlying channel access mechanism: contention-based, contention-free, and low power listening (LPL) or polling. The following subsections will provide details with their pros and cons.

2.2.1 Contention-Based MAC Protocols

Sensor nodes contend for shared medium using contention-based channel access mechanism to communicate with other nodes or coordinator. Unavailability of predefined schedule for communication results in variable latency and packet loss. CSMA is a contention-based mechanism to access available shared medium for data transmission. CSMA/CA is a modification of CSMA algorithm to avoid packet collision. Ready to send (RTS) and clear to send (CTS) are used in CSMA before packet transmission; however, in CSMA/CA without RTS/CTS exchange, before transmission

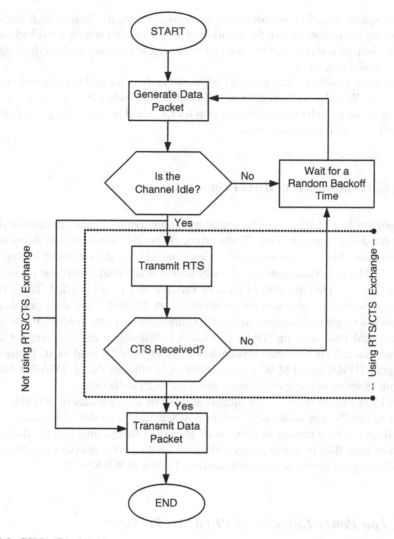

Fig. 2.1 CSMA/CA algorithm

of data packets, nodes listen to shared medium/channel to find out whether shared channel is idle or not. In case of idle situation, node starts transmission of data packets. However, if channel is sensed busy, transmission is rescheduled for a random period of time. Figure 2.1 shows CSMA/CA simplified algorithm.

To ensure reliable and collision-free communication, a common schedule is used with contention called as scheduled contention. In some cases, we need a schedule-based contention channel access mechanisms called as scheduled contention. A common schedule is used for data communication to ensure reliability and collision avoidance. Scheduled-contention mechanisms required periodic synchronization. To maintain synchronization, schedules are exchanged on regular basis which leads to extra energy consumption. Synchronization of nodes is highly sensitive to clock drift. Periodic sleep of nodes in this mechanism reduces idle listening and overhearing to improve power efficiency.

Contention-based mechanisms are well suited in dynamic and scalable networks. However, in WBANs such mechanisms do not provide reliable and efficient communication due to high energy consumption for CCA and poor handling capabilities for emergency and on-demand traffic.

2.2.2 Contention-Free MAC Protocols

In contention-free MAC protocols, sensor nodes are assigned guaranteed time slots (GTS) for data communication. These protocols provide deterministic delay with no packet loss due to communication in guaranteed time slots without contention period. TDMA is a contention-free channel access mechanism where the channel is divided into multiple time slots of fixed or variable length, see Fig. 2.2. These time slots are allocated to end nodes for communication. Multiple time slots can also be assigned to a single node depending upon requirements and data volume. Predefined and dedicated time slots in TDMA provide a collision-free environment for data communication. Synchronization is the key issue in TDMA-based MAC protocols. In general, TDMA-based MAC protocols are more efficient than CSMA/CA-based protocols in terms of energy efficiency and bandwidth utilization.

TDMA is a suitable option for limited number of sensor nodes in WBANs with fixed data rate. Sensor nodes only wake up in specified time slots for communication; otherwise, they remain in sleep mode to avoid idle listening and overhearing. Assigning time slots to sensor nodes with different data rates, nonperiodic data, and scalability are the key issues in implementing TDMA in WBANs.

2.2.3 Low Power Listening (LPL) MAC Protocols

In LPL mechanism, sensor nodes periodically listen to the channel. Nodes go into sleep mode if the channel is sensed idle; otherwise, keep the transceiver in active mode to receive data packets. This mechanism is also known as "Polling." In polling-

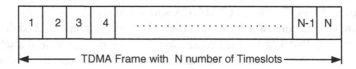

Fig. 2.2 TDMA frame structure

based MAC protocol, time interval is divided into an idle interval and wakeup interval. During the idle interval, ordinary nodes sleep to avoid extra power consumption due to idle listening [6].

Once the idle interval ends, all nodes wake up to listen the long preamble transmitted by the network coordinator. The preamble contains the address of the polled node. Once the node receives the preamble with its address, either it transmits the data packet or the null packet indicating that the buffer of the node is empty. LPL mechanisms avoid idle listening and overhearing. Synchronization is not required here. Due to hardware complexity and listening of long preamble, LPL mechanisms are not well suited to WBANs. LPL mechanisms support simplex communication. However, WBANs require duplex channel communication to accommodate periodic, on-demand, and emergency traffic.

2.3 MAC Protocols for WBAN

Many researchers have proposed various MAC protocols for WBAN. Some of them have been submitted to Task Group 6, which was formed in 2007 to address the problems/issues of WBAN and to define relevant standards. Due to the similarity of WBAN and WPAN, most proposed protocols are based on superframe structure of IEEE 802.15.4. However, time-critical communication and high QoS requirements are needed for WBAN, for which IEEE 802.15.4 falls in short. To achieve the QoS requirements for time-critical application of WBANs, a number of protocols that are not based on IEEE 802.15.4 have been proposed so far [7–15]. This section covers the pros and cons of some of these prominent MAC protocols proposed for WBANs. The protocols are introduced with emphasis on energy consumption and how they tackle energy inefficiency caused by collision, overhearing, idle listening, and control packet overhead.

2.3.1 Battery-Aware TDMA Protocol

Battery-aware TDMA protocol [7] is one of the protocols designed for WBANs to maximize the lifespan of the network using cross-layer approach. A number of parameters are considered to design this protocol, which include: time-varying wireless fading channel, electrochemical properties of battery, and packet queuing characteristics. Periodic beacons are transmitted by the coordinator just as IEEE 802.15.4 does. The time axis is divided into three time slots: (1) active time slot, (2) inactive period, and (3) beacon slot. Figure 2.3 shows the frame structure of this protocol.

To support different applications of WBANs, the frame structure is adaptive and can be changed. Periodic wakeup mechanism is introduced to avoid idle listening of nodes. A dedicated time slot T_s is assigned to each node, where data is transmitted by end node when it receives beacon from the coordinator. Dedicated GTS assigned

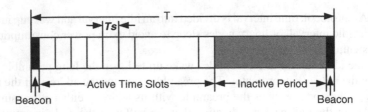

Fig. 2.3 Frame structure of battery-aware TDMA protocol

to each node improves reliability and timely delivery of packets. End nodes remain in sleep mode for the inactive period of time to avoid extra consumption of energy. However, the lack of mechanism to accommodate emergency data and holding of data packets in buffer for long intervals are the two drawbacks of this proposed solution. In addition, packet buffering might result in high packet delay and packet drop rate.

2.3.2 Priority-Guaranteed MAC Protocol

Superframe structure plays an important role in the design of MAC protocols. A new superframe structure is introduced for the priority-guaranteed MAC protocol [8], as shown in Fig. 2.4. Time axis is divided into two main portions: active and inactive periods. Active time period is further divided into five parts to accommodate various kinds of data flow. Control Channel AC1 and Control Channel AC2 are used for uplink control of life-critical medical applications and consumer electronics applications, respectively. Two different times slots are reserved for period and burst data known as Time Slot Reserved for Periodic traffic (TSRP) and Time Slot Reserved for Burst traffic (TSRB), respectively. Beacon is used for synchronization on nodes. For uplink control, randomized ALOHA is used by AC1 and AC2. However, TDMA is used to assign GTS to end nodes for data communication in the two data channels. The performance of this mechanism is better than IEEE 802.15.4 in terms of energy consumption. Unadaptability to emergency data traffic and complexity of superframe are the major shortcomings.

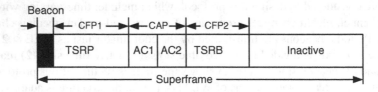

Fig. 2.4 Superframe structure of priority-guaranteed MAC

2.3.3 Energy-Efficient Low Duty Cycle MAC Protocol

Energy-efficient Low Duty Cycle (ELDC) is one of the TDMA-based protocols proposed to accommodate streaming of large amount of data [9]. Network life is maximized with efficient utilization of TDMA approach for medium access. In the proposed network topology, master node (MN) is responsible for on-body network coordination and synchronization. The time axis is divided into multiple time slots, as shown in Fig. 2.5. End nodes are assigned dedicated time slots S1 to Sn. To facilitate the communication of emergency/on-demand traffic, time slots RS1 and RS2 are reserved. Acceptable packet drop, packet error rate, and number of sensor nodes are the parameters used to decide the number of reserved channels for on-demand traffic.

Guard band time slots are inserted between two consecutive time slots to avoid overlapping/collision of data transmission caused by clock drifts. To facilitate simultaneous data communications from end nodes and to MS (monitoring station), MN uses two transceivers with different physical layer communication models. ELDC performs better in terms of energy efficiency, high data rate, and accommodation of short burst of data. However, period synchronization will cause extra energy consumption.

Two types of communication models can be employed in this context. First, MN has one transceiver. In this case, enough time is reserved for communication of MN with MS. In the second case, where the MN has two transceivers, simultaneous communication of MN with MS and sensor nodes is possible. The communication uses different physical layer communication models for transparency. Due to features of pure TDMA and fixed frame structure, the protocol fails to accommodate on-demand traffic.

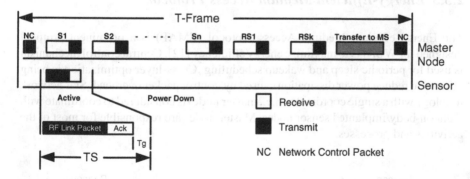

Fig. 2.5 Frame structure of ELDC

2.3.4 A Power-Efficient MAC Protocol for WBANs

In [10] researchers have proposed a power-efficient MAC Protocol to accommodate the normal, on-demand, and emergency traffic in WBANs. Two wakeup mechanisms are introduced to improve the network performance for not only normal traffic but also for on-demand and emergency data traffic. The data traffic generated by routine monitoring of physiological is categorized as normal traffic. In life-critical applications, some of the in/on or around the human body sensor nodes initiate emergency traffic. End nodes are requested by coordinator for on-demand traffic to acquire information if needed. To accommodate all these three types of communication patterns, the time axis in superframe is divided into three parts: a beacon message, a configurable contention access Period (CCAP) to accommodate short burst of data where slotted ALOHA is used for channel access, and a contention-free period (CFP) where GTS are assigned to end nodes for collision-free communication. The newly defined superframe structure is shown in Fig. 2.6.

Traffic-based wakeup table is maintained by the coordinator for different applications. Unnecessary energy dissipation is controlled by periodic sleep/wakeup mechanism. Sensor nodes wake up in advance for time interval of $T_K = 2\theta T_W$ in order to compensate clock drift either at coordinator or end node; T_W is the beacon period. Wakeup radio signals are sent from end node to coordinator and coordinator to end node for emergency and on-demand traffic, respectively. This protocol performs better than WiseMAC [11]. However, low power listening is not an optimal solution for improved efficiency in on-body or implanted sensor nodes.

2.3.5 Energy-Efficient Medium Access Protocol

The Energy-efficient Medium Access Protocol (EMAP) is a prominent protocol designed for WBANs to maximize energy efficiency [12]. Central control mechanism is used for periodic sleep and wakeup scheduling. Cross-layer optimization is being utilized to reduce power dissipation caused by control packet overhead. Star network topology with a single coordinator (i.e., master node) is considered to coordinate with eight on-body/implanted sensor nodes. Master nodes are responsible for most of the activities and processes.

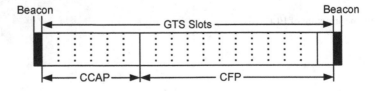

Fig. 2.6 Superfame structure of power-efficient MAC protocol

The operation is based on three processes: link establishment, sleep/wakeup scheduling, and exception process. Link establishment occurs when a node wants to join the cluster. Nodes are assigned unique scheduling for sleep and wakeup periods to communicate with master node. This procedure helps to avoid extra energy consumption due to idle listening and overhearing. Exception process is initiated to facilitate communication of emergency data. Wakeup Fallback Time (WFT) is introduced to make the communication guaranteed and reliable. In case of data communication failure in specific wakeup interval, the sensor node enters a sleep interval defined by WFT. This mechanism helps to avoid overlapping of time slots.

It is observed from the simulation results of different physiological signs that the power consumption depends upon the number of retransmissions and sleep intervals. Centrally-controlled idle listening and overhearing reduce energy consumption efficiently. However, there are some limitations in implementation which include, e.g., complexity, limited number of nodes in a cluster, lack of mechanism for on-demand data, and link establishment process where only one node can establish a link at a time.

2.3.6 BodyMAC

TDMA is one of the most reliable and widely used channel access mechanism for WBANs. BodyMAC utilizes the TDMA channel access mechanism to define uplink and downlink subframes to improve power efficiency [13]. End nodes use periodic sleep scheduling when they have no data to communicate. *Burst Bandwidth procedure, Periodic Bandwidth procedure, and Adjust Bandwidth procedure* are the three procedures used to accommodate different data streaming. Improved network stability and control packet transmission are achieved with this flexible and efficient bandwidth management.

As shown in Fig. 2.7, MAC frame is divided into three parts: beacon, downlink, and uplink. Beacons are used for periodic synchronization whereas downlink is used for communication from coordinator to end node for on-demand traffic. The uplink frame is divided into Contention Access Period (CAP) and CFP for different kind of

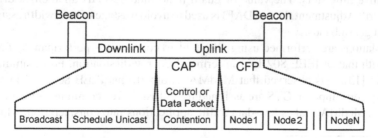

Fig. 2.7 Superframe structure for BodyMAC

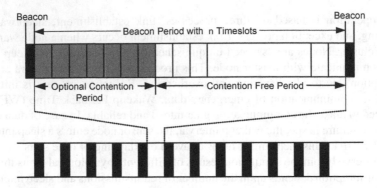

Fig. 2.8 Superframe with m Beacons for MedMAC

services. Communication in CAP is based on CSMA/CA where small data packets
and control requests for guaranteed time slots are sent to coordinator. Sensor nodes
are assigned guaranteed time slots for communication in CFP, which improve the
performance in terms of energy consumption. However, CCA and packet collision
in CAP result in high energy consumption.

2.3.7 MedMAC

MedMAC [14] is one of the TDMA-based proposed protocols for WBANs to improve
power efficiency and channel access. This protocol utilizes the TDMA approach to
assign GTS to end nodes. However, the GTS assigned by this protocol are of variable
length and depend on the applications. A novel mechanism with multisuperframe
is used for periodic synchronization, as show in Fig. 2.8. An optimum contention
period is used for network initialization, emergency traffic, and low data streaming.

Timestamp scavenging with Adaptive Guard Band Algorithm (AGBA) is introduced by MedMAC to maintain clock synchronization of coordinator and end nodes.
Packet collision is avoided with unique GTS assignment and synchronization of
nodes using AGBA. A guard band time defined by AGBA is inserted between two
consecutive time slots. The value of guard band time depends upon clock drift of
nodes. Drift Adjustment Factor (DAF) is used to avoid wastage of bandwidth assigned
for extra guard bands.

Simulations are performed using OPNET[1] to compare the performance of Med-
MAC with that of IEEE 802.15.4 in terms of energy dissipation. From simulation
results in [13], it is observed that MedMAC outperforms IEEE 802.15.4 in terms
of energy consumption. GTS are assigned for collision-free communication of data.
However, MedMAC takes low-data traffic applications into consideration, which is

---

[1]OPNET is a simulation tool used for performance analysis of computer networks and applications.
Details can be found at https://www.opnet.com/.

not always applicable in WBANs where data rates for in/on or around the human body sensor nodes may be high.

2.3.8 Heartbeat-Driven MAC Protocol

Heartbeat-Driven is a TDMA-based protocol which utilizes heartbeat rhythm for synchronization [15]. Like some of the previously mentioned protocols, this protocol uses a star network topology with GTS allocation for collision-free data communication. heartbeat rhythm is used instead of periodic control messages for network synchronization required by TDMA mechanism. Information of heartbeat rhythm are extracted from sensory data by each biosensor node for synchronization. The coordinator is responsible to assign time slots to individual nodes and calculate the number of frame cycles for synchronization.

Idle listening and overhearing are controlled with synchronized communication in dedicated time slots. Utilizing heartbeat rhythm for synchronization reduces the power consumption. However, heartbeat rhythm cannot be available to all in/on or around the human body sensor nodes. In such cases, it is difficult to synchronize with the system. On the other hand, complexity increases if the sensor nodes without heartbeat rhythm information are integrated with other sensor nodes.

2.4 Discussion

Energy efficiency is one the most important goals to be achieved in CPS like WBAN. Healthcare applications over WBAN include data streaming of critical and noncritical physiological signs sensed by in/on or around the human body sensor nodes. It has been the focus of researchers to improve the performance of WBAN in terms of reliability and energy efficiency at the MAC layer. However, other techniques including, e.g., cross-layer approach, antenna design, and RF communication and propagation models also affect the performance of WBAN. Mobility, transparency, interoperability, security, and high QoS are the other main issues to be considered by researchers for improved and high-quality healthcare services outside as well as inside the hospitals.

Multiple medium access techniques have been used at MAC layer for shared medium access. The prominent four techniques are CSMA, TDMA, FDMA, and CDMA. Selection of medium access technique depends upon application and hardware compatibility. CDMA is the best option for channel access where packet collision is not acceptable. This is not a suitable choice in WBAN due to limited computational and power capabilities of sensor nodes. Similarly, hardware complexity required for FDMA to avoid collision in WBAN makes it an inappropriate choice for channel access. For dynamic networks like WBAN, CSMA outperforms in terms of reliable communication and low delay. However, protocol overhead and extra energy consumption for channel assessment are the major shortcomings of CSMA. TDMA is the best approach for guaranteed communication, but this approach also faces some issues, including, e.g., synchronization, nonadaptability, and scalability. Based on limited numbers of sensor nodes in WBANs, TDMA could be considered the suitable channel access approach. A number of MAC protocols, based on these observations, have been proposed so far to improve reliability and power efficiency in WBANs. However, efforts are still needed to develop protocols to avoid energy dissipation due to collision, overhearing, and idle listening with reduced control packet overhead and implementation complexities. Other design objectives include high bandwidth utilization, fairness at MAC layer, minimum delay, reliable communication, and reduced synchronization cost. Furthermore, the protocols should also have the capabilities to accommodate communication of normal, emergency, and on-demand traffic generated by different in/on or around human body sensor nodes.

2.5 Summary

In this chapter, existing MAC protocols for CPS like WBAN are introduced with emphasis on energy minimization. These protocols have been developed to prolong lifespan of the system, reliable communication, flexibility, fair management, and QoS. MAC protocols based on random access and LPL are unable to accommodate emergency and on-demand traffic. On the other hand, TDMA-based protocols can potentially improve the performance of WBANs. Consequently, the majority of existing MAC protocols for WBANs are based on TDMA approach. Each of them have some advantages and disadvantages. Due to diverse application requirements and hardware constrains, none of them has been accepted as a standard. New protocols need to be developed to address requirements of WBANs like energy efficiency, scalability, fairness, reduced implementation complexity, support for diverse applications, interoperability, reduced synchronization overhead, and QoS.

References

1. Rahim A, Javaid N, Aslam M, Rahman Z, Qasim U, Khan ZA (2012) Comprehensive survey of MAC protocols for wireless body area networks. In: Seventh international conference on broadband and wireless computing, communication and applications (BWCCA). doi:10.1109/BWCCA.2012.77
2. IEEE-802.15.4a-2007. Part 15.4: wireless medium access control (MAC) and physical layer (PHY) specifications for low-rate wireless personal area networks (LR-WPANs): amendment to add alternate PHY. Standard, IEEE
3. Doudou M, Djenouri D, Badache N, Bouabdallah A (2014) Synchronous contention-based MAC protocols for delay-sensitive wireless sensor networks: a review and taxonomy. J Netw Comput Appl. doi:10.1016/j.jnca.2013.03.012

4. Thotahewa KMS, Redoute JM, Yuce MR (2004) Medium access control (MAC) Protocols for ultra-wideband (UWB)-based wireless body area networks (WBAN). Ultra-wideband and 60 GHz communications for biomedical applications. doi:10.1007/978-1-4614-8896-5_7
5. 802.15.6-2012 - IEEE standard for local and metropolitan area networks—part 15.6: Wireless body area networks. Standard, IEEE
6. Misic VB, Misic J (2014) A polling MAC for wireless sensor networks with RF recharging of sensor nodes. In: 7th Biennial symposium on communications (QBSC). doi:10.1109/QBSC.2014.6841188
7. Su H, Zhang X (2009) Battery-dynamics driven TDMA MAC protocols for wireless body-area monitoring networks in healthcare applications. IEEE J Sel Areas Commun. doi:10.1109/JSAC.2009.090507
8. Zhang Y, Dolmans G (2009) A new priority-guaranteed MAC protocol for emerging body area networks. In: Fifth international conference on wireless and mobile communications. doi:10.1109/ICWMC.2009.30
9. Marinkovic SJ, Popovici EM, Spagnol C, Faul S, Marnane WP (2009) Energy-efficient low duty cycle MAC protocol for wireless body area networks. IEEE Trans Inf Technol Biomed. doi:10.1109/TITB.2009.2033591
10. Ameen MA, Liu J, Ullah S, Kwak KS (2011) A power efficient MAC protocol for implant device communication in wireless body area networks. In: 2011 IEEE consumer communications and networking conference (CCNC). doi:10.1109/CCNC.2011.5766358
11. El-Hoiydi A, Decotignie JD (2004) WiseMAC: an ultra low power MAC protocol for the WiseNET wireless sensor network. Algorithm Asp Wirel Sens Netw. doi:10.1007/978-3-540-27820-7_4
12. Omeni O, Wong ACW, Burdett AJ, Toumazou C (2008) Energy efficient medium access protocol for wireless medical body area sensor networks. IEEE Trans Biomed Circuits Syst. doi:10.1109/TBCAS.2008.2003431
13. Fang G, Dutkiewicz E (2009) BodyMAC: energy efficient TDMA-based MAC protocol for wireless body area networks. In: 9th international symposium on communications and information technology. doi:10.1109/ISCIT.2009.5341045
14. Timmons NF, Scanlon WG (2009) An adaptive energy efficient MAC protocol for the medical body area network. In: 1st international conference on wireless communication, vehicular technology, information theory and aerospace & electronic systems technology. doi:10.1109/WIRELESSVITAE.2009.5172512
15. Li H, Tan J (2010) Heartbeat-driven medium-access control for body sensor networks. IEEE Trans Inf Technol Biomed. doi:10.1109/TITB.2009.2028136

Chapter 3
Evaluating IEEE 802.15.4 for CPS

Abstract This chapter provides a brief introduction of IEEE 802.15.4 and its compatibility toward CPS. IEEE 802.15.4 was not designed for networks that provide guaranteed QoS, while the performance of cyber-physical applications usually depends highly on QoS of the underlying networks. Therefore, it becomes necessary and important to assess the applicability of IEEE 802.15.4 protocol in CPS. Here the performance of IEEE 802.15.4 is analyzed in beacon-enabled and non-beacon-enabled modes, respectively. The network QoS is characterized by several metrics, including effective data rate, packet loss rate, and end-to-end delay. These metrics are examined with respect to different MAC parameter settings.

Keywords Quality of Service · Network analysis · Protocol · Network simulator · Synchronization

3.1 Introduction

The rapid developmental growth of CPS has not only attracted the academia and industry but also the government institutions. So far, many conferences, workshops, and summits have been held to discuss the opportunities and challenges brought by CPS which is generally built upon WSANs, an extension of WSNs. In this context, WSANs are generally responsible for information exchange (i.e., data transfer), serving as a bridge between the cyber and the physical worlds [1–3]. For this purpose, the IEEE 802.15.4 protocol [4] has been utilized in a lot of CPS applications over WSANs. Despite the wide popularity of IEEE 802.15.4 networks, their applicability to CPS needs to be validated [5, 6]. This is because IEEE 802.15.4 was not designed for networks that can provide QoS guarantees, while the performance of cyber-physical applications often depends highly on the QoS of underlying networks.

Since the release of IEEE 802.15.4 in 2003, in order to characterize the performance of this standard, a number of simulation and analytical studies have been presented [7, 8]. However, most of these studies mainly focus on IEEE 802.15.4 in either the beacon-enabled mode or non-beacon-enabled mode. For instance, the performance of IEEE 802.15.4 has been evaluated in beacon-enabled mode using NS-2[1] [9]. Analytical Markov model is used to evaluate the performance and behavior of IEEE 802.15.4 slotted CSMA/CA mechanism [10]. The slotted CSMA/CA mechanism of IEEE 802.15.4 is studied for performance evaluation using enhanced Markov chain models [11]. Beacon Order and Superframe Order parameters are analyzed in beacon-enabled mode of IEEE 802.15.4 [12, 13]. Under different topological organizations, a flexible mathematical model has been presented in [14] to study the performance of beacon-enabled IEEE 802.15.4. With respect to different configurable environments, different traffic loads and different scenarios, the performance of non-beacon-enabled IEEE 802.15.4 has been evaluated [15–20]. In addition, IEEE 802.15.4 has also been evaluated for special applications, e.g., WSN, WBAN, and emergency response [21–29].

This chapter reports our work [3, 30] on analyzing the performance of IEEE 802.15.4 protocol in both beacon-enabled and non-beacon-enabled modes based on a one-hop star network, using the OMNeT++[2] simulator. End-to-end delay, effective data rate, and packet loss rate are the three QoS metrics which are analyzed with respect to different protocol parameters. In-depth analysis of the results provides insights for adapting IEEE 802.15.4 for CPS. By analyzing the results, IEEE 802.15.4 can be easily configured and optimized for enhanced performance in CPS.

3.2 IEEE 802.15.4

IEEE 802.15.4 is a standard designed for low-rate PANs [4]. It covers the PHY layer and the MAC layer specifications. PHY layer is defined for the operation in three different unlicensed ISM frequency bands, which includes 27 communication channels. This protocol operates in two different modes: beacon-enabled mode and non-beacon-enabled mode. In beacon-enable mode, the coordinator sends beacon frames periodically. The beacon interval defines time between two consecutive beacon frames. It contains an active period and optionally, an inactive period. The active period is also called as superframe, which is divided into 16 equal time slots. The superframe contains a beacon frame, a CAP, and a CFP. During the CAP, a CSMA/CA mechanism is used for data transmission. The CFP is optional and contains up to 7 GTSs in each superframe. GTS are reserved for specified nodes to transmit time-critical packets.

---

[1]Network Simulator (NS) is a specialized discreet event simulation tool for TCP, routing, and multicast protocols over wired and wireless networks. http://www.isi.edu/nsnam/ns/.

[2]OMNeT++ is component-based C++ framework used for network simulations with modular and extension capabilities; URL: http://www.omnetpp.org/.

Table 3.1 IEEE 802.15.4 frequency bands and modulation

Frequency (MHz)	Frequency band (MHz)	Data rate (kbps)	Modulation scheme
868	868–868.6	20	BPSK
915	902–928	40	BPSK
2400	2400–2483.5	250	O-QPSK

3.2.1 Overview

As mentioned previously, IEEE 802.15.4 defines PHY and MAC sublayer. PHY layer is defined for operation in three different unlicensed ISM frequency bands (i.e., 2.4 GHz band, 915 MHz band, and 868 MHz band), which includes 27 communication channels in total. An overview of modulation schemes and frequency bands used by IEEE 802.15.4 is given in Table 3.1.

There are two different kinds of devices defined in IEEE 802.15.4: Full Function Device (FFD) and Reduced Function Device (RFD). An FFD can act as an ordinary device or a PAN coordinator. But RFD can only serve as a device supporting simple operations. An FFD can communicate with both RFDs and other FFDs, while an RFD can only communicate with FFDs.

IEEE 802.15.4 supports a star topology or a peer-to-peer topology. In star networks, all the communications are between end devices and the sink node which is also called PAN coordinator. The PAN coordinator manages the whole network, including distributing addresses to the devices and managing new devices that join in. In the peer-to-peer network, the devices can communicate with any other devices which are within their range of signal radiation. A specific type of peer-to-peer networks is cluster tree networks. In this case, most of the devices are FFD.

3.2.2 MAC Sublayer

To interact with the PHY layer, MAC sublayer handles physical radio channel access. MAC layer is responsible for the following features and tasks.

- Beacon management
- Synchronization of network devices
- Channel access
- Association and disassociation
- Frame validation and acknowledgements
- GTS management
- Peer-to-peer link establishment.

Conceptually, for layer management and services interfaces, MAC sublayer consists of a management entity, called MLME. The MAC data service enables to transmit and receive MAC Protocol Data Units (MPDUs).

3.2.3 Superframe Structure

The IEEE 802.15.4 standard supports two kinds of network configuration modes:

- Beacon-enabled mode: A Personal Area Network (PAN) coordinator periodically generates beacon frames after every Beacon Interval (BI) in order to identify its PAN to synchronize with associated nodes and to describe the superframe structure.
- Non-beacon-enabled mode: All nodes can send their data by using an unslotted CSMA/CA mechanism, which does not provide any time guarantee to deliver data frames.

In beacon-enabled mode, the coordinator node transmits beacon frames periodically in order to achieve synchronization of attached device, PAN identification and to describe superframes' structure. A superframe is always bounded by two consecutive beacons and may consist of an active period and an optional inactive period, as shown in Fig. 3.1. All communications must take place during the active part. In the inactive part, devices can be powered down/off to conserve energy.

The active part of the superframe is divided into 16 equally sized slots and consists of 3 parts: a beacon, a CAP, and an optional CFP. The beacon shall be transmitted at the start of slot 0 without the use of CSMA/CA, and the CAP shall commence immediately after the beacon and complete before the beginning of CFP on a superframe slot boundary.

The superframe structure is described by two parameters: Beacon Order (BO) and Superframe Order (SO). Both parameters can be positive integers between 0 and 14. The values of BO and SO are used to calculate the length of the superframe

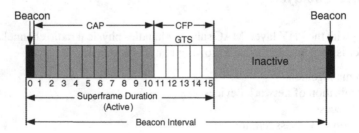

Fig. 3.1 Superframe structure

(i.e., Beacon Interval, *BI*) and its active period (i.e., Superframe Duration, *SD*) respectively, as defined as follows:

$$BI = aBaseSuperframeDuration \times 2^{BO}$$
$$SD = aBaseSuperframeDuration \times 2^{SO}$$
$$DutyCycle = SD/BI = 2^{SO-BO}$$

where aBaseSuperframeDuration is a constant, representing the number of symbols forming a superframe when *SO* is equal to 0. The *BO* and *SO* must satisfy the relationship $0 \leq SO \leq BO \leq 14$. According to the IEEE 802.15.4 standard, the superframe will not be active anymore if $SO = 15$. Moreover, if $BO = 15$ the superframe shall not exist and the non-beacon-enabled mode will be used. The relationship between *BI* and *SD* is used to define duty cycle.

3.2.4 Contention Access Period (CAP)

In beacon-enabled mode, nodes willing to communicate compete for channel access in CAP between the two beacons transmitted by coordinator. Beacon is transmitted at the start of slot 0 and CAP starts immediately after the beacon and ends before the beginning of CFP. The available CAP portion provides scalability and flexibility for new or other network devices to join. All the transactions and communication are completed using CSMA/CA mechanism.

3.2.5 Contention Free Period (CFP)

In order to accommodate low latency applications or to provide specific data bandwidth to applications, GTS are assigned by coordinator in CFP which starts after CAP and finishes at the end of active superframe. Up to 7 GTS slots can be assigned by coordinator and more than one time slot may be occupied by a single GTS. Communication of each device in CFP should be completed one IFS period before the end of its GTS.

3.2.6 Inter Frame Spacing (IFS)

The received data needs a finite time to be processed at MAC layer. An IFS period is used to separate the two successive frames transmitted by a device. However, if the first transmission needs an acknowledgment, the second transmission should wait for an IFS after receiving the acknowledgment. The duration of IFS depends upon the size of frame that has just been transmitted. A frame is followed by Short

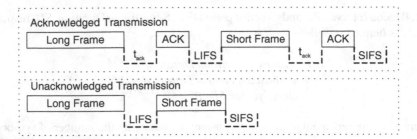

Fig. 3.2 Interframe spacing

Interframe Spacing (SIFS) if the frame size is up to *aMaxSIFSFrameSize* octets, otherwise followed by Long Interframe Spacing (LIFS) if the frame size is greater than *aMaxSIFSFrameSize* octets. In CAP, CSMA/CA follows this mechanism for data transmission. Figure 3.2 illustrate the concepts of LIFS and SIFS.

3.2.7 CSMA/CA Mechanism

As mentioned above, CSMA/CA is used before transmission of MAC or data frames in CAP. It is not used for beacon transmission in beacon-enabled mode. In addition, it is not used for MAC, data, or acknowledgement frames in CFP. If the periodic beacon-enabled mode is used for communication in PAN, slotted CSMA/CA is used for communication in CAP. However, unslotted CSMA/CA is used in non-beacon-enabled mode for channel access.

In both cases, the CSMA/CA algorithm is implemented based on backoff periods, where one backoff period will be equal to a constant, known as *aUnitBackoffPeriod*. Transmissions are synchronized with beacon if slotted CSMA/CA is used. The first backoff period of each superframe starts with the transmission of the beacon, and the backoff will resume at the start of the next superframe if it has not been completed at the end of the CAP. In contrast, in the case of unslotted CSMA/CA, the backoff periods of devices are not related in time to other devices. Three variables are maintained by each device for frame transmission.

In the CSMA/CA algorithm each device in the network has three variables: *NB*, *CW*, and *BE*. To attempt for transmission of current frame, the required numbers of backoff are presented by *NB*. Before initiating a new transmission, the value of *NB* is initially set to zero. *CW* is only used in slotted CSMA/CA, representing the number of backoff period to be cleared before starting of a new transmission. However, to count the number of backoff periods a device should wait for before initiating transmission is counted by *BE*. Figure 3.3 illustrates step by step CSMA/CA algorithm.

For unslotted CSMA/CA, *NB* and *BE* are initialized before step 2. In slotted CSMA/CA, *CW NB* and *BE* are initialized and boundary of next backoff period is located in step 1. In slotted CSMA/CA, CCA starts on backoff period boundary.

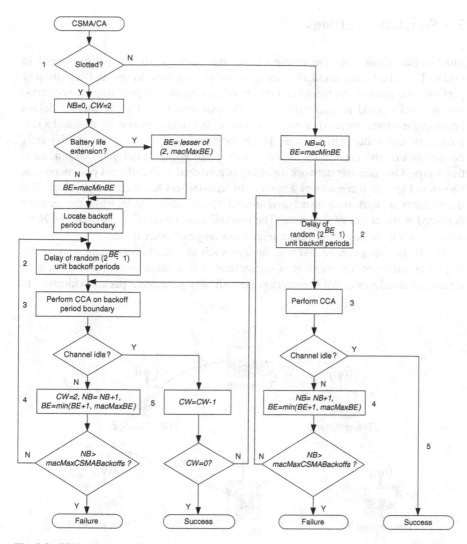

Fig. 3.3 CSMA/CA algorithm

CCA starts immediately in unslotted CSMA/CA after $random(2^{NB} - 1)$ unit backoff periods. MAC sublayer increments both *NB* and *BE* by one, if the channel is found to be busy, ensuring that *BE* should not be more than *macMaxBE*. *CW* is also assigned the value of 2. Channel access failure occurs if the value of *NB* is greater than *macMaxCSMABackoffs*, otherwise CSMA/CA algorithm proceeds to step 2.

If the channel is found idle, in unslotted CSMA/CA, transmission of frame is started by MAC sublayer immediately. In slotted CSMA/CA, to ensure that contention window has expired before initiating transmission, MAC sublayer first decrements *CW* by one and then transmits if *CW* is equal to zero; otherwise proceeds to step 3.

3.3 Simulation Settings

This section deals with the configuration and settings for simulation model in OMNeT++, including simulation scenario and parameter settings, and definition of performance metrics. As mentioned previously, compared to peer-to-peer networks, star networks could be preferable for CPS applications and yield smaller delays because the communication in star networks occurs only between devices and a single central controller, while any device in the peer-to-peer networks can arbitrarily communicate with each other as long as they are within a common communication range. One-hop star network topology is analyzed with different parameters, as shown in Fig. 3.4. It consists of a number of transmitters and a central receiver. The transmitters are uniformly distributed around a 50 m radius circle, while the receiver is placed at the center of the circle. The transmission range of every node is 176 m, where every node lies with in communication range of other node.

The transmitters can be taken as devices such as sensors communicating to the central coordinator. The number of transmitters will change with scenarios in non-beacon-enabled mode. All transmitters periodically generate a packet addressed to

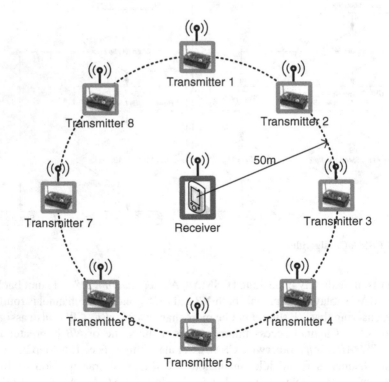

Fig. 3.4 Simulated network topology. Reprinted from Ref. [3]

the receiver. In the PHY layer, 2.4 GHz spectrum is used with a data rate of 250 kbps. To analyze the performance several variable parameters are selected to be examined, which may have significant influence on the performance of IEEE 802.15.4, including MAC Service Data Unit (MSDU) size, packet generation interval, *MaxNB*, *MinBE*, and *MaxFrameRetries* in non-beacon mode, and *MaxNB*, *BO*, and *SO* in beacon-enabled mode. Some important fixed parameters and default values of variable parameters are listed in Table 3.2.

The performance of network protocols for CPS needs to be real-time, reliable, and resource efficient [5, 6]. In order to meet these requirements, end-to-end delay, effective data rate, and packet loss rate are selected as QoS metrics.

(i) End-to-End Delay: It is a crucial metric to evaluate the real-time performance of networks. It refers to the average time difference between the points when a packet is generated at the network device (transmitter) and when the packet is received by the network coordinator (receiver).

Table 3.2 Simulation parameters

Parameter	Value
Carrier frequency	2.4 GHz
Transmitter power	1 mW
Carrier sense sensitivity	−85 dBm
Transmission range	176 m
Bit rate	250 Kbps
Traffic type	Exponential
Number of packets sent by every device (in non-beacon-enabled mode)	5000
Run time (in beacon-enabled mode)	1000 s
MaxBE	5
MinBE	3 (default)
MaxNB	4 (default)
MaxFrameRetries	3 (default)
MAC payload size (MSDU size)	60 Bytes (default)
Packet generation interval (in non-beacon-enabled mode)	0.025 s(default)
Packet generation interval (in beacon-enabled mode)	0.05 s
Superfame order (SO) (in beacon-enabled mode)	6 (default)
Beacon order (BO) (in beacon-enabled mode)	7 (default)
Number of devices (in beacon-enabled mode)	8

Reprinted from Ref. [3]

(ii) Effective Data Rate: It is an important metric to evaluate the link bandwidth utilization which reflects the resource efficiency as well as dependability of networks. It is defined as below:

$$RefData = \frac{N_{susspacket} \times L_{MSDU}}{T_{end} - T_{start}}$$

where $N_{susspacket}$ is the total number of usable data packets which are received successfully by coordinator from all devices in the simulation time. L_{MSDU} is the MSDU length of the data frame. $T_{end} - T_{start}$ is the total time of the transmission from the beginning to the end.

(iii) Packet Loss Rate: It indicates the performance of reliability. It is the ratio of the number of packets dropped by the network to the total number of packets generated at all devices. From the above definitions, it is clear that the effective data rate is closely related with packet loss rate. Higher packet loss rate leads to lower effective data rate for the same number of transmitters.

3.4 Non-beacon-Enabled Mode

This section presents the impact of five impact factors (i.e., MSDU size, packet generation interval, *MaxNB*, *MinBE*, and *MaxFrameRetries*) on the performance of IEEE 802.15.4 networks in terms of the above-mentioned metrics, respectively. During simulation process, when a specific parameter is examined as the impact factor, other parameters are assigned default values.

3.4.1 Impact of MSDU Size

MSDU size is the payload size of MAC layer frame and its maximum size is 128 bytes. Figure 3.5 depicts the measured effective data rate, which increases with MSDU size for the same number of transmitters.

Reduced overhead with respect to the same number of nodes with maximum MSDU size increases data efficiency. It is observed that for a given MSDU size, when the number of transmitters increases, the effective data rate first increases and then decreases. This is due to the fact that with increase in the number of transmitters, packet collision increases with increasing number of packets. At the beginning, with less contention for the medium, effective data rate increases; however, with increase in contention due to increased number of transmitters, effective data rate reduces.

As the number of transmitters increases, contention probability increases. In such case the packet loss will normally increase. As shown in Fig. 3.6, the measured packet loss rate for the same MSDU size is increasing with increase in the number of transmitters. Since the bandwidth capacity is limited and increase in MSDU will lead

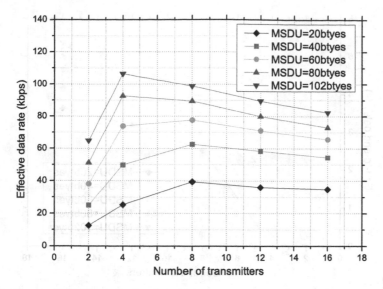

Fig. 3.5 Impact of MSDU on effective data rate

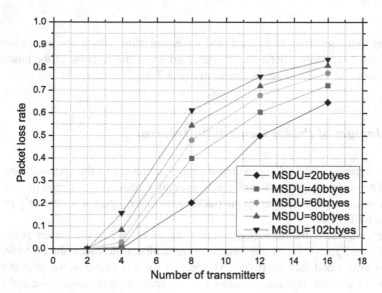

Fig. 3.6 Impact of MSDU on packet loss rate

to higher data transmission rate, with increase in MSDU size for a certain number of transmitters the probability of packet loss will increase, as shown in the Fig. 3.6.

Figure 3.7 depicts the measured end-to-end delay. The curve trend in the figure is similar to that in Fig. 3.6. From the above analysis of packet loss rate, it is clear that more transmitters and larger MSDU sizes increase the probability of packet collision.

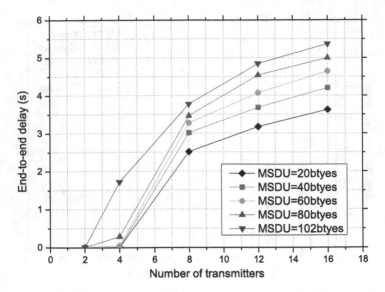

Fig. 3.7 Impact of MSDU on end-to-end delay

This can increase times of backoff and retransmission, which are a considerable factor for longer delay. Therefore, the delay grows as the increase of the number of transmitters and MSDU size, as shown in Fig. 3.7.

3.4.2 Impact of Packet Generation Interval

All transmitters periodically generate a packet addressed to the receiver. The time interval between the generation of two consecutive packets is referred to as packet generation interval. It is apparent the packet generation interval is inversely proportional to traffic load.

Figure 3.8 shows the measured effective data rate. When the packet generation interval is less than 0.1 s, as the number of transmitters increases, the effective data rate first grows and then decreases. The reason for this phenomenon is that as the number of transmitters increases, more packets are sent in the same time and traffic load increases; but overly heavy traffic load leads to higher possibility of collision which causes the decrease of the effective data rate. On the other hand, when the interval is larger than 0.1 s, although the number of transmitters increases, the traffic load is still very low. This is the reason why the effective data rate always keeps increasing as the number of transmitters increases.

Figure 3.9 illustrates the measured packet loss rate, which is lower when the packet generation interval is larger than 0.1 s. This is because larger packet generation intervals imply lighter traffic load and hence less collisions happen. On the other

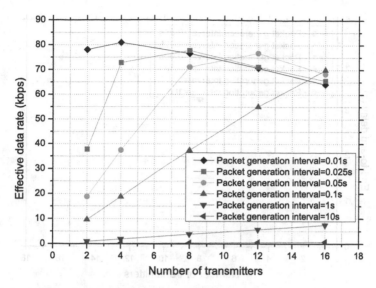

Fig. 3.8 Impact of packet generation interval on effective data rate

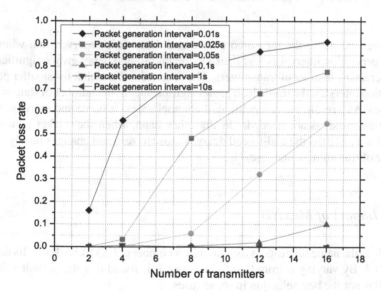

Fig. 3.9 Impact of packet generation interval on packet loss rate

hand, when the packet generation interval is less than 0.1 s, for a given small packet generation interval, the packet loss rate increases with the number of transmitters. In the meantime, for a certain number of transmitters, the packet loss rate increases as the interval decreases. This could be explained that smaller packet generation intervals mean heavier traffic load which increases the probability of packet collision.

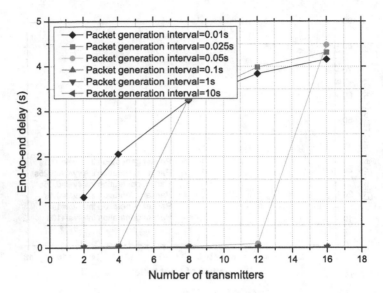

Fig. 3.10 Impact of packet generation interval on end-to-end delay

Figure 3.10 shows the measured end-to-end delay. It is observed that when the packet generation interval is less than 1 s, the end-to-end delay grows significantly with increasing number of transmitters. The reason for this is that for smaller packet generation intervals, the traffic load grows significantly as the number of transmitters increases. As a result, the competition of channel access is fierce and more backoffs and retransmissions are needed. On the other hand, when the packet generation interval is 1 s or 10 s, the end-to-end delay is close to zero and changes hardly as the number of transmitters increases.

3.4.3 Impact of MaxNB

MaxNB, as the name suggests, is the maximum number of CSMA backoffs. Its default value is 4. By varying it from 0 to 5, however, it is found that the default value of *MaxNB* is not the best selection in some cases.

Figure 3.11 indicates that the measured effective data rate increases as the value of *MaxNB* increases in case of limited number of transmitters. However, when the number of transmitters reaches a certain threshold, the situation becomes opposite, as shown in the Fig. 3.11. It is observed that effective data rate decreases with increasing value of *MaxNB* for dense networks.

In Fig. 3.12, for the same number of transmitters, contrary to the effective date rate in Fig. 3.10, the packet loss rate decreases for less transmitters with the increase of

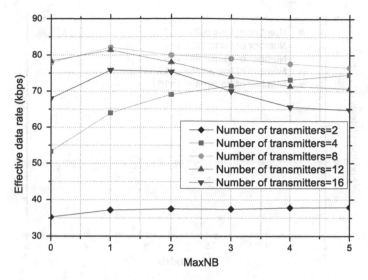

Fig. 3.11 Impact of MaxNB on effective data rate

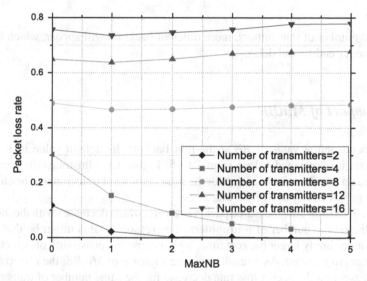

Fig. 3.12 Impact of MaxNB on packet loss rate

MaxNB. Nevertheless, when the number of transmitters reaches a certain threshold, the situation becomes opposite.

Figure 3.13 depicts the measured end-to-end delay, which is close to 0 for less (e.g., 2 or 4) transmitters as shown in the figure. This is due to the fact that for less transmitters, the channel is often idle and few collisions happen. On the other hand, for more transmitters, the delay grows with increasing *MaxNB*. This is because with

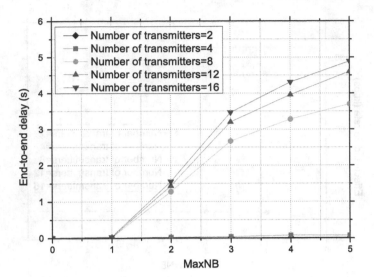

Fig. 3.13 Impact of MaxNB on end-to-end delay

increased number of transmitters, more times of backoffs will appear, which in turn lead to longer end-to-end delay.

3.4.4 Impact of MinBE

MinBE is the initial value of *BE* at the first backoff. Its default value is 3. In the simulations it is assigned values from 1 to 5. Figure 3.14 illustrates the measured effective data rate. It is observed that for the same number of transmitters, the effective data rate grows slowly as MinBE increases.

Figure 3.15 shows the measured packet loss rate, which decreases with the increase of *MinBE* and the number of transmitters. The reason for this might be that larger *MinBE* values imply larger backoff time, which cause the possibility of detecting an idle channel to increase. As a result, with the increase of *MinBE*, the effective data rate increases and the packet loss rate decrease for the same number of transmitters.

Figure 3.16 shows the measured end-to-end delay. With the same number of transmitters, the end-to-end delay grows with the increase of *MinBE*.

3.4.5 Impact of MaxFrameRetries

MaxFrameRetries refers to the maximum times of retransmission. If the retransmission times of a packet exceed the *MaxFrameRetries* value, it will be discarded.

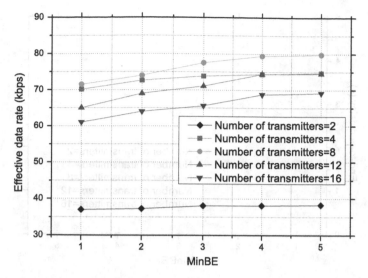

Fig. 3.14 Impact of MinBE on effective data rate

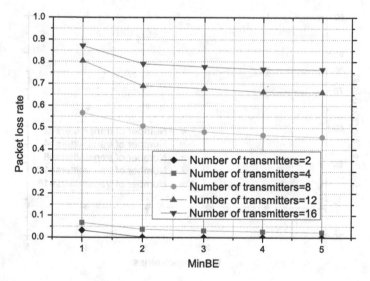

Fig. 3.15 Impact of MinBE on packet loss rate

Simulations are performed with different values of *MaxFrameRetries* from 0 to 5. Figure 3.17 shows the measured effective data rate in this regard. For a given larger number of transmitters, the effective data rate decreases slightly with the increase of *MaxframeRetries*, while it increases for less transmitters.

In Fig. 3.18, for the same number of transmitters the curve trend of packet loss rate is opposite to that of effective data rate in Fig. 3.17. The reason behind this is similar to that of the *MaxNB* analysis. Figure 3.19 shows the measured end-to-end delay.

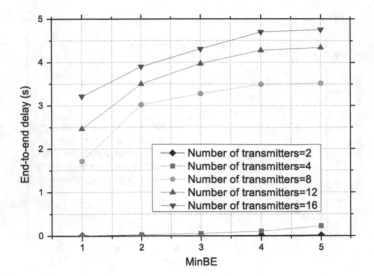

Fig. 3.16 Impact of MinBE on end-to-end delay

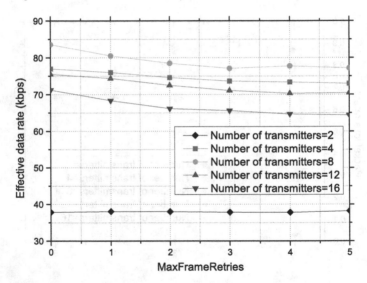

Fig. 3.17 Impact of MaxFrameRetries on effective data rate

It is perceived that for less transmitters, the channel is often idle. Consequently, most of the frames can be transmitted successfully for the first time. As a result, the delay is close to 0. However, as the number of transmitters increases, the network load becomes heavier and the possibility of collision increases. Many packets need to be retransmitted for more times. This leads to the fact that end-to-end delay grows with the increase of *MaxFrameRetries* for the more transmitters.

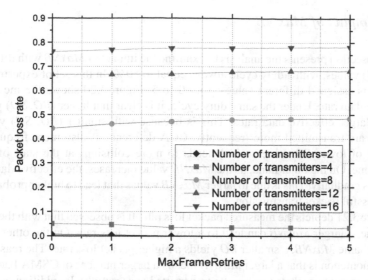

Fig. 3.18 Impact of MaxFrameRetries on packet loss rate

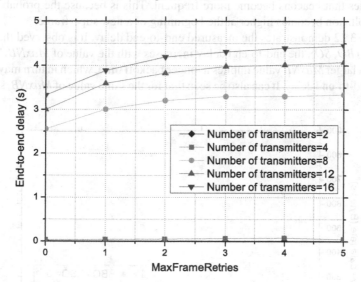

Fig. 3.19 Impact of MaxFrameRetries on end-to-end delay

3.5 Beacon-Enabled Mode

This section presents the performance analysis of IEEE 802.15.4 in beacon-enabled mode. Simulations are carried out to examine how *MaxNB*, *SO*, and *BO* affect the network QoS with IEEE 802.15.4 standard.

3.5.1 Impact of MaxNB

This subsection presents the analysis to examine the impact of *MaxNB* with different (BO, SO) values, with a duty cycle always equal to 50%. In this set of experiments, *MaxNB* is assigned different values from 0 to 5. Figure 3.20 shows the measured effective data rate. Under the same duty cycle, it is clear that larger (BO, SO) values lead to larger effective data rates. This is because with smaller (BO, SO) values, beacons are transmitted more frequently. CCA deference is also more frequent in the case of lower SO values, which leads to more collisions at the start of each superframe. On the other hand, as the *MaxNB* value increases, the effective data rate increases gradually. This is due to larger *MaxNB* values that lead to higher probability of successful packet transmission.

Figure 3.21 depicts the measured packet loss rate. It is observed that with the same BO value, a larger *MaxNB* can lead to a lower packet loss rate. On the other hand, with the same *MaxNB*, a smaller BO yields a higher packet loss rate. The reason for this phenomenon is that a larger *MaxNB* means a larger number of CSMA backoffs, resulting in more packets that can be transmitted successfully. In addition, a lower BO implies that beacons become more frequent. This is because the probability of packet collision becomes higher at the beginning of a new superframe.

Figure 3.22 demonstrates the measured end-to-end delay. It is observed that with the same (BO, SO), the end-to-end delay increases with the value of *MaxNB*. This is because a larger *MaxNB* value implies a longer backoff time, which in turn may cause longer end-to-end delay. It can also be seen that for the same value of *MaxNB*, smaller

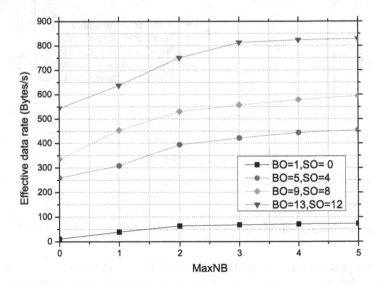

Fig. 3.20 Impact of MaxNB on effective data rate

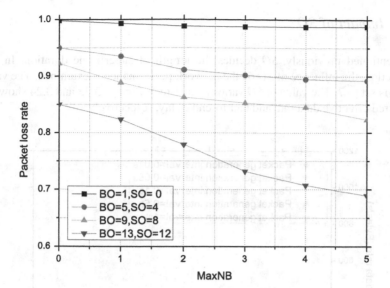

Fig. 3.21 Impact of MaxNB on packet loss rate

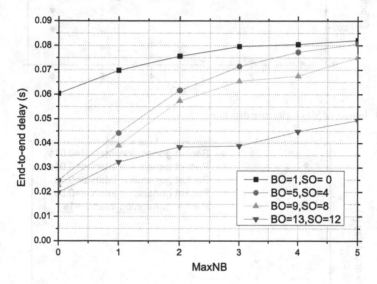

Fig. 3.22 Impact of MaxNB on end-to-end delay

average delay can be obtained with larger (*BO*, *SO*) values. This is mainly due to the less packet collisions and retransmissions, which has been explained previously.

3.5.2 *Impact of SO*

As mentioned previously, *SO* decides the length of superframe duration. In this Subsection, the influence of *SO* on the network performance is examined. The value of *BO* is set to 7. The value of *SO* varies from 1 to 6. Figures 3.23 and 3.24 show the measured effective data rate and end-to-end delay, respectively.

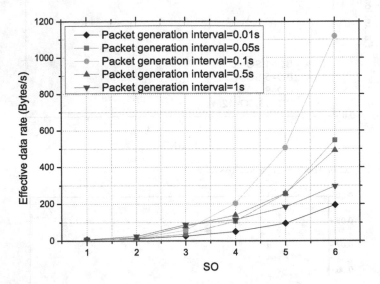

Fig. 3.23   Impact of SO on effective data rate

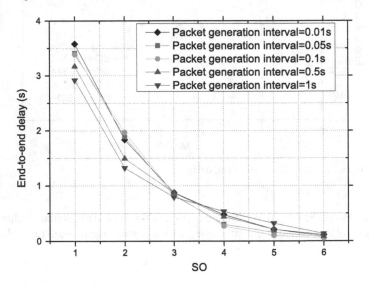

Fig. 3.24   Impact of SO end-to-end delay

For the same packet generation interval, a larger *SO* with the same *BO* achieves a higher effective data rate and a lower end-to-end delay. This is because a larger *SO* implies a longer active period with a higher duty cycle. As a result, the network has a better ability to transmit packets within current superframe, and hence less packets will experience a long sleeping delay.

Figure 3.25 depicts the measured packet loss rate. It can be seen that with the same packet interval, a larger *SO*, which implies a higher duty cycle, yields a lower packet loss rate. When the packet interval is 0.01 s, the packet loss rate is almost 100 % all the time. The reason behind this is that with a larger *SO*, more packets can be transmitted within the current superframe. On the other hand, with the same *SO*, the packet loss rate decreases as the packet generation interval increases.

3.5.3 Impact of BO

In this subsection, the influence of *BO* is examined that how it affects network performance. The value of *BO* controls the length of superframe (i.e., beacon interval). First, *SO* is assigned value of 1 and then network performance is evaluated with different *BO* values from 7 to 2.

Figure 3.26 shows the measured effective data rate. It is observed that as the value of *BO* decreases, effective data rate grows gradually. This is mainly because the smaller *BO* resulting in higher duty cycle can achieve larger bandwidth, which implies larger effective data rates.

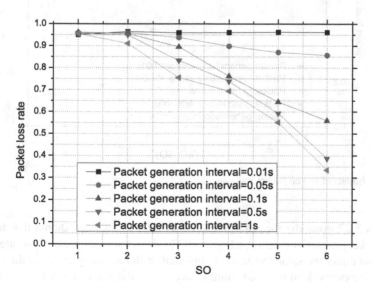

Fig. 3.25 Impact of SO on packet loss rate

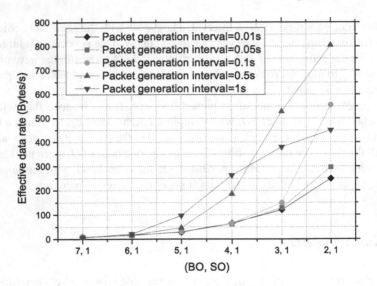

Fig. 3.26 Impact of BO on effective data rate

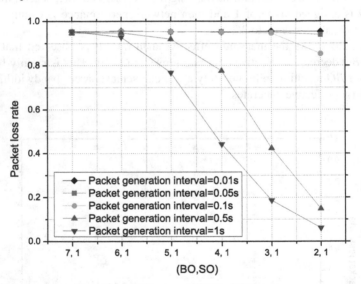

Fig. 3.27 Impact of BO on packet loss rate

Figure 3.27 gives the measured packet loss rate. It has been shown that for the same packet generation interval, a higher *BO* leads to a smaller packet loss rate. This is because under the same traffic load, the smaller *BO* resulting in larger duty cycle enables the network to transmit more packets. For the same *BO*, when the traffic load decreases, the packet loss rate descends from top (nearly 100 %) to a very small value. This effect can be explained as follows: a smaller packet generation interval

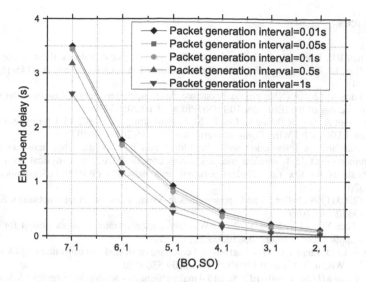

Fig. 3.28 Impact of BO on end-to-end delay

implies a higher traffic load and hence more packets need to be retransmitted as a result of collisions.

Figure 3.28 presents the measured end-to-end delay. It is clear that higher delays are experienced for larger *BO* values with the same packet generation interval. The reason is that a larger *BO* causes a longer inactive period, in which case buffered packets may potentially experience a longer sleeping delay. For the same *BO*, the increase in packet generation interval results in decreased average delay. This is easy to understand since heavier traffic loads as a consequence of smaller packet generation intervals may cause more collisions and retransmissions.

3.6 Summary

In this chapter, comprehensive performance evaluation of IEEE 802.15.4 standard is presented with respect to two different modes in the context of CPS. Considering general requirements of CPS applications, several network QoS metrics including effective data rate, packet loss rate, and end-to-end delay have been examined. These metrics are analyzed with respect to some important and variable protocol parameters. The analysis of simulation results provides some insights for configuring and optimizing the IEEE 802.15.4 protocol for CPS applications. A key finding is that the default configuration specified in the standard may not yield the best QoS in all cases. Consequently, some protocol parameters should adapt to the environments, while taking into account the CPS application requirements.

References

1. Rajkumar RR, Lee I, Sha L, Stankovic J (2010) Cyber-physical systems: the next computing revolution. In: Proceedings of the 47th design automation conference. doi:10.1145/1837274. 1837461
2. Poovendran R (2010) Cyber physical systems: close encounters between two parallel worlds. In: Proceedings of the IEEE. doi:10.1109/JPROC.2010.2050377
3. Xia F, Vinel A, Gao R, Wang L, Qiu T (2011) Evaluating IEEE 802.15.4 for cyber-physical systems. EURASIP J Wirel Commun Netw. doi:10.1155/2011/596397
4. IEEE standard for information technology-local and metropolitan area networks-specific requirements-part 15.4: wireless medium access control (MAC) and physical layer (PHY) specifications for low rate wireless personal area networks (WPANs). September 2006, pp 1–320
5. Xia F (2008) QoS challenges and opportunities in wireless sensor/actuator networks. Sensors. doi:10.3390/s8021099
6. Xia F, Tian YC, Li Y, Sung Y (2007) Wireless sensor/actuator network design for mobile control applications. Sensors. doi:10.3390/s7102157
7. Wang, F, Li D, Zhao Y (2009) Analysis and compare of slotted and unslotted CSMA in IEEE 802.15.4. WiCom'09. doi:10.1109/WICOM.2009.5303580
8. Zheng J, Lee MJ (2004) Will IEEE 802.15.4 make ubiquitous networking a reality? A discussion on a potential low power, low bit rate standard. IEEE Commun Mag 42:140–146
9. Lu G, Krishnamachari B, Raghavendra CS (2004) Performance evaluation of the IEEE 802.15.4 MAC for low-rate low-power wireless networks. In: 2004 IEEE international conference on performance, computing, and communications. doi:10.1109/PCCC.2004.1395158
10. Pollin S, Ergen M, Ergen S, Bougard B, Der Perre L, Moerman I, Bahai A, Varaiya P, Catthoor F (2008) Performance analysis of slotted carrier sense IEEE 802.15.4 medium access layer. IEEE Trans Wirel Commun. doi:10.1109/TWC.2008.060057
11. Jung CY, Hwang HY, Sung DK, Hwang GU (2009) Enhanced Markov chain model and through-put analysis of the slotted CSMA/CA for IEEE 802.15.4 under unsaturated traffic conditions. IEEE Trans Veh Technol. doi:10.1109/TVT.2008.923669
12. Huang YK, Pang AC, Hung HN (2009) A comprehensive analysis of low-power operation for beacon-enabled IEEE 802.15.4 wireless networks. IEEE Trans Wirel Commun. doi:10.1109/TWC.2009.081485
13. Ren S, Aung KMM, Park JS (2006) A probe for the performance of low-rate wireless personal area networks. Intell Control Autom. doi:10.1007/978-3-540-37256-1_21
14. Buratti C (2010) Performance analysis of IEEE 802.15.4 Beacon-enabled mode. IEEE Trans Veh Technol. doi:10.1109/TVT.2010.2040198
15. Kim TO, Park JS, Chong HJ, Kim KJ, Choi BD (2008) Performance analysis of IEEE 802.15.4 non-beacon mode with the unslotted CSMA/CA. IEEE Commun Lett. doi:10.1109/LCOMM. 2008.071870
16. Buratti C, Verdone R (2008) A mathematical model for performance analysis of IEEE 802.15.4 non-beacon enabled mode. In: Wireless conference. doi:10.1109/EW.2008.4623881
17. Latre B, Mil PD, Moerman I, Dhoedt B, Demeester P, Dierdonck NV (2006)Throughput and delay analysis of unslotted IEEE 802.15.4. J Netw. doi:10.4304/jnw.1.1.20-28
18. Rohm D, Goyal M, Hosseini H, Divjak A, Bashir Y (2009) A simulation based analysis of the impact of IEEE 802.15.4 MAC parameters on the performance under different traffic loads. Mob Inf Syst. doi:10.3233/MIS-2009-0074
19. Rohm D, Goyal M, Hosseini H, Divjak A, Bashir Y (2009) Configuring beaconless IEEE 802.15.4 networks under different traffic loads. In: International conference on advanced infor-mation networking and applications. doi:10.1109/AINA.2009.84
20. Buratti C, Verdone R (2009) Performance analysis of IEEE 802.15.4 non beacon-enabled mode. IEEE Trans Veh Technol. doi:10.1109/TVT.2009.2014956
21. Howitt I, Gutierrez JA (2003) IEEE 802.15.4 low rate-wireless personal area network coexis-tence issues. Wirel Commun Netw. doi:10.1109/WCNC.2003.1200605

22. Salles N, Krommenacker N, Lecuire V (2008) Performance study of IEEE 802.15.4 for industrial maintenance applications. In: IEEE international conference on industrial technology. doi:10.1109/ICIT.2008.4608681
23. Chen F, Wang N, German R, Dressler F (2010) Simulation study of IEEE 802.15.4 LR-WPAN for industrial applications. Wirel Commun Mob Comput. doi:10.1002/wcm.736
24. Liang X, Balasingham I (2007) Performance analysis of the IEEE 802.15.4 based ECG monitoring network. In: Proceedings of the 7th IASTED international conferences on wireless and optical communications. ACTA, Montreal
25. Li C, Li H B, Kohno R (2009) Performance evaluation of IEEE 802.15.4 for wireless body area network (WBAN). In: ICC workshops 2009. doi:10.1109/ICCW.2009.5208087
26. Liu J, Demirkiran I, Yang T, Helfrick A (2009) Feasibility study of IEEE 802.15.4 for aerospace wireless sensor networks. In: Digital avionics systems conference. doi:10.1109/DASC.2009.5347576
27. Chen F, Talanis T, German R, Dressler F (2009) Real-time enabled IEEE 802.15.4 sensor networks in industrial automation. In: IEEE international symposium on industrial embedded systems. doi:10.1109/SIES.2009.5196207
28. Mehta A, Bhatti G, Sahinoglu Z, Viswanathan R, Zhang J (2009) Performance analysis of beacon-enabled IEEE 802.15.4 MAC for emergency response applications. In: Proceedings of the 3rd international conference on advanced networks and telecommunication systems. doi:10.1109/ANTS.2009.5409873
29. Zen K, Habibi D, Rassau A, Ahmad I (2008) Performance evaluation of IEEE 802.15.4 for mobile sensor networks. In: International conference on wireless and optical communications. networks. doi:10.1109/WOCN.2008.4542536
30. Gao R, Xia F, Wang L, Qiu T, Vinel A (2011) Performance analysis of non-beaconed IEEE 802.15.4 for high-confidence wireless communications. In: Baltic conference on future internet communications. doi:10.1109/BCFIC-RIGA.2011.5733221

Chapter 4
IEEE 802.15.4 Based Adaptive MAC Protocols

Abstract WSANs provide the infrastructure for many applications of CPS. Lots of these applications use the IEEE 802.15.4 standard. However, it does not provide any means of differentiated services to improve QoS for time-critical and delay-sensitive events. A large amount of efforts have been made to address such issues. In this chapter, an overview on some interesting mechanisms used in existing adaptive and real-time protocols in compliance with IEEE 802.15.4 is presented. Careful examination of these research works reveals that by optimizing the original specifications and dynamically adjusting the protocol parameters, the total network efficiency can be significantly improved. Nevertheless, there are still certain challenges to overcome in pursuing the most appropriate protocol without introducing unacceptable side-effects.

Keywords ZigBee · Guaranteed communication · Contention window · Scheduling · Protocol design

4.1 Introduction

WSANs built upon IEEE 802.15.4 [1] constitute the communication infrastructure of various CPS applications. Examples of these applications include large-scale factory automation [2], distributed and process control [3, 4], machinery health monitoring [5–7], among many others. IEEE 802.15.4 and ZigBee specification [8] provide the specifications from physical layer to application layer in communication stack. These standards have greatly encouraged to bridge the real-time physical world's applications/objects to cyber world for diverse range of time-critical applications. The communication and computing capabilities of cyber core are utilized to control/monitor real world's objects/applications.

The performance of CPS depends upon QoS of the underlying network. In practice, applications' requirements vary in different environments. For example, in case of environmental surveillance, alarm packet should be prioritized as compared to normal data readings. In WBANs, life critical physiological readings should be delivered on time to the health services provider. However, IEEE 802.15.4 does not have such

© The Author(s) 2015
F. Xia and A. Rahim, *MAC Protocols for Cyber-Physical Systems*,
SpringerBriefs in Computer Science, DOI 10.1007/978-3-662-46361-1_4

mechanism to differentiate or accommodate time-critical information over the network. In addition, bandwidth requirement varies for different nodes in a network. For example, a node in WBAN to monitor ECG requires more bandwidth as compared to a node monitoring body temperature. IEEE 802.15.4 stands in need of proper mechanism to deal with such requirements for data communication [9].

In order to achieve guaranteed QoS for different applications of CPS, many researchers have been attracted to address timeliness, adaptivity, and flexibility to improve the performance and to prolong the life-span of CPS applications [10–12]. Based on IEEE 802.15.4, lots of protocols have been proposed so far to accommodate the requirement of each node to perform real-time computations and to send high-quality data with guaranteed QoS [13–18]. In this chapter, which is based on our previous work [19], we present an overview on some interesting mechanisms used in existing adaptive and real-time protocols based on IEEE 802.15.4.

4.2 Approaches for Contention Access Period

To access the shared medium, slotted CSMA/CA mechanism is used by IEEE 802.15.4 in CAP. IEEE 802.15.4 does not provide any mechanism for differentiated service, e.g., to accommodate time-critical data streaming like fire alarm or critical physiological signs. In CPS, some nodes might send data more frequently as compared to normal communication. In such cases, with standard slotted CSMA/CA approach for shared channel it is hard to achieve network efficiency with respect to different bandwidth requirements of end nodes. In fact, it has been observed [20–30] that IEEE 802.15.4 does not perform well to achieve adaptivity and real-time guaranteed communication in dense networks where a number of nodes contend for shared channel access.

The four parameters which are initialized and significantly affect the behavior of slotted CSMA/CA are: (1) the minimum backoff exponent $macMinBE$, (2) the maximum backoff exponent $aMaxBE$, (3) the initial value of CW CW_{init}, and (4) the maximum number of backoffs $macMaxCSMABackoff$.

The two parameters, $macMinBE$ and $aMaxBE$, are often set to default values, respectively. These values are used to provide a range for random selection of backoffs in order to access the shared medium. Network performance changes when one of these or both values are changed. For example, if the BE value is decremented to a value less than the default value 3, the lower boundary of the possible backoff value will decrease consequently. This results in reduced waiting time to access the channel when the shared medium is detected busy or packet collision occurs. CCA is performed more frequently with reduced waiting time, increasing the possibility of successful transmission. Throughput performance increases significantly as compared to nodes where CCA requires a longer waiting time.

It is observed in [9] that the initial value of $macMinBE$ does not affect the network throughput performance for large-scale WSAN (or WSN). However, the impact of $macMinBE$ on the network throughput is quite important in small-scale networks.

The throughput of network decreases with increasing value of *macMinBE*. Due to efficient collision avoidance, the probability of successful transmission increases.

CW_{init}, the initial value of CW, is another parameter for IEEE 802.15.4 that is useful to differentiate transmission of packets in slotted CSMA/CA. This parameter presents the number of CCAs performed prior to packet transmission to monitor whether the medium is busy or idle.

In order to protect the ACK frame and giving enough time for receiving node to process the frame, IEEE 802.15.4 defines that the transmitter should perform CCA twice. The receiver should send the ACK frame after time t_{ACK} if it is acquired by the transmitter. t_{ACK} varies from 12 to 31 symbols (one backoff period is 20 symbols). Hence, one-time of CCA can potentially cause a collision between a newly transmitted packet and an ACK packet. Nevertheless, one-time of CCA gives a strong priority to obtain the channel. For a backoff counter, the range of the counter drawn for a high-priority packet's backoff procedure should be bounded by a smaller constant value than a normal packet's in order to enable a faster transmission. Provided that ACK collision is not so severe, the flexible CW value will definitely guarantee a better rate of successful transmission for a device with high priority as compared to conventional IEEE 802.15.4 MAC protocol, where every device initiates the CCA procedure with the same CW.

Performance of IEEE 802.15.4 is also affected by the parameter *macMaxCSMA Backoff*, which represents the maximum number of times the CSMA/CA algorithm is required to backoff while attempting to access the channel. In an ideal communication environment, nearly all undelivered packets are dropped by the protocol because they exceed the maximum number of backoff stages (i.e., *macMaxCSMABackoff*). In this way, a larger *macMaxCSMABackoff* which means a larger number of CSMA backoffs can result in more packets that can be transmitted successfully and lead to a lower packet loss rate. It is observed from simulation results in [24] that increasing the *macMaxCSMABackoff* parameter, while leaving all other parameters to their default values, results in an almost linear increase in the delivery ratio. The end-to-end delay will increase with the value of *macMaxCSMABackoff*. This is because a larger *macMaxCSMABackoff* value implies a larger number of packets is successfully transmitted, which takes a longer backoff time, and in turn may cause longer end-to-end delay.

The low-efficiency problem originated by CSMA/CA algorithm at MAC layer is made worse by default parameters settings. Previous performance evaluation [29] shows that the default parameters setting is inappropriate for most of applications. Hence, the key question to answer is whether a more appropriate parameter setting can solve the problem without introducing unacceptable side-effects. Recently, a wide variety of parameter tuning approaches in CAP have been proposed to improve network efficiency.

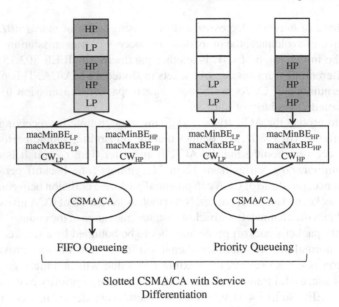

Fig. 4.1 Differentiated service strategies. Reprinted from ref. [19]

4.2.1 Adaptive Backoff Exponent Mechanism

The service differentiation mechanism proposed in [13] is particularly based on *macMinBE* and *aMaxBE* parameters. Based on importance of data traffic and command frames, the command frames are prioritized higher as compared to data frames. Thus the traffic is classified into two subclasses: low priority and high priority. Figure 4.1 presents the differentiated service strategies.

This algorithm assigns different attributes to both classes and changes the CSMA/CA parameters instead of having the same for both classes of data. Backoff interval and contention window initial values for high-priority data are presented by *macMinBE$_{HP}$*, *macMaxBE$_{HP}$* and *CW$_{HP}$*, while for low priority data transfer these values are presented by *macMinBE$_{LP}$*, *macMaxBE$_{LP}$* and *CW$_{LP}$*.

By setting *CW$_{HP}$* higher than *CW$_{LP}$*, low priority traffic has to assess the channel to be idle for a longer time before transmission. On the other hand, providing lower backoff delay values for high-priority traffic by setting *macMinBE$_{HP}$* lower than *macMinBE$_{LP}$* will improve its responsiveness without degrading its throughput.

In addition to the specification of different CSMA/CA parameters, priority queuing is applied to reduce queuing delays of high-priority traffic. In this case, slotted CSMA/CA uses priority scheduling to select frames from queues, and then applies the adequate parameters corresponding to each service class.

This differentiated service scheme for slotted CSMA/CA in IEEE 802.15.4 serves to improve the performance of time-sensitive messages. It has been shown that tuning

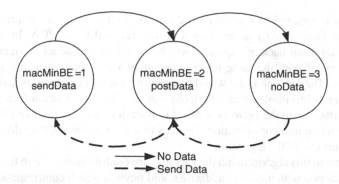

Fig. 4.2 State transition scheme. Reprinted from ref. [19]

adequately the *BE* parameter of slotted CSMA/CA may result in an improved quality of service for time-critical messages.

A new State Transition Scheme (STS) is additionally proposed in [20]. By adjusting the *macMinBE* value of some nodes to a smaller value and by dynamically changing the value depending on the transmission conditions, the scheme can shorten the backoff delay of nodes with frequent transmission.

In the MAC modifications, the value of the *macMinBE* is a number between 1 and 3, which changes flexibly as the condition of the node changes. As seen in Fig. 4.2, each node has three states, *noData*, *postData*, *sendData*, with each state having the default *macMinBE* value of 3, 2, and 1, respectively.

In the STS, the three states are switched dynamically and nodes are requested to count the number of idle beacon frames (with no transmission) and the number of successful transmissions within a beacon frame, before the CCA process. By counting the numbers, we can allow the nodes with more data to transmit to a higher priority in the network. The STS will not make additional fairness problems because if a node has nothing to send any more it increases the *macMinBE* so that it can be excluded from the high-priority nodes.

The change lets the modified node take advantage in transmitting data as compared to the nonmodified nodes, causing higher throughput performance for the modified node. By implementing the STS, the throughput performance of the overall network is significantly improved.

Also in this line, Rao and Marandin presented a brief study of the CSMA/CA mechanism in [25], with emphasis on the improper *BE* distribution which results in frequent packet collisions and a loss in systems performance. They provided an algorithm called the adaptive backoff exponent (ABE) which reduces the probability of devices choosing identical number of backoff periods at collision rates, thus improving the system's performance considerably at these rates.

The ABE algorithm is primarily based on three important principles. The first is the idea of providing a higher range of backoff exponents to the devices so as to reduce the probability of devices choosing the same number of backoff periods to sense the channel. The second is to do away with a constant minimum back-off exponent (*macMinBE*) value as used in the standard CSMA/CA. In this algorithm, the minimum backoff exponent will be variable, and hence devices are not likely to start off with the same backoff exponent when they wish to start a data transmission. The last one is the way the minimum backoff exponent is maintained. Since the algorithm implements a variable *macMinBE*, the variation factor is each node's contribution to the network traffic. Only devices that are involved in a transmission are taken into consideration. Devices that are not transmitting do not come under the purview of the algorithm.

According to this algorithm, all devices that are contributing more to the network traffic are slapped with higher *macMinBEs*, and devices which contribute less to the network congestion will use lower minimum backoff exponents. Therefore, devices with higher *macMinBE* values are likely to wait longer than devices with lower *macMinBEs*, leading to an overall improvement in effective data bandwidth.

4.2.2 Adaptive Contention Window Mechanism

A frame tailoring (FRT) strategy is proposed in [26] to avoid ACK and data packet collision while allowing one-time CCA it can be exploited to provide strong prioritization in addition to the standard CSMA/CA.

In this scheme, the length of t_{ACK} is determined as depicted in Fig. 4.3, depending on packet length, and the term frame tail is defined as the length of the remainder after the total packet length is divided by the backoff slot length (i.e., 20 symbols). If a frame tail is from 0 to 8 symbols, a receiver transmits an ACK packet at the very next backoff slot boundary as depicted in Fig. 4.3a, b. On the other hand, if a frame tail ranges from 9 to 19 symbols, an ACK transmission by the receiver is postponed to one backoff slot after the next backoff slot boundary to allow adequate time to prepare the ACK transmission. As a result, t_{ACK} becomes more than 20 symbols as shown in Fig. 4.3c. Then, the CCA operations of other contending nodes during this time interval report that the medium is idle. To protect ACK transmissions in such cases, two-time CCAs are mandated in IEEE 802.15.4 slotted CSMA/CA. FRT strategy is to adjust each data packet length so that t_{ACK} becomes exactly 12 symbols as shown in Fig. 4.3b. By doing so, one-time CCA will never declare an idle medium during the time period between a data and an ACK, and hence by adopting one-time CCA for a particular transmission, high prioritization can be achieved.

The proposed FRT strategy effectively separates the medium access of each group of packet transmissions according to packet's priority. By adopting the proposed scheme, the probability of transmission deferment to the next active period due to competitive contention is relaxed and bounded delay is provided to high-priority packets.

Kim and Kang proposed a mechanism of contention window differentiation (CWD) in [27] to provide multilevel differentiated services for IEEE 802.15.4 sensor

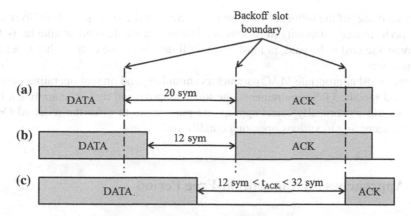

Fig. 4.3 Variable t_{ACK} depending on data packet length. Reprinted from ref. [19]

networks. CWD is a mechanism assigning various values of CW according to the priority classes. Let $class0, \ldots, classQ$ be the set of priority classes ordered by

$$classQ \prec class(Q-1) \prec \cdots \prec class0 \qquad (4.1)$$

where $\prec$ denotes the order of priority. Equation (4.1) implies that $class0$ and $classQ$ are the highest and lowest priority classes, respectively. They differentiate the corresponding CW value of priority $classQ$ by $CW[Q]$ as follows:

$$CW[0] \leq CW[1] \leq \cdots \leq CW[Q] \qquad (4.2)$$

The relationship in (4.2) is intuitive, since a device with a smaller CW has a better chance of transmission than a device with a larger CW in general. In other words, a device with high priority can start transmission when a device with low priority is performing the CCA procedure. It guarantees a better rate of successful transmission for a device with high priority compared with the conventional 802.15.4 MAC protocol, where every device initiates the CCA procedure with the same CW.

Numerical results show that the IEEE 802.15.4 standard in WSNs can support adaptive and timely packet transmissions by tuning the MAC parameters to more appropriate values. However, the increase in reliability is usually achieved at the cost of a higher latency, and high adaptivity and low delay may demand a significant energy consumption and network complexity, thus making a great many approaches not feasible at best. Due to the random nature of CSMA/CA algorithm, an appropriate parameters setting which guarantees both adaptivity and bounded latency for real-time applications is hardly achieved. There are also other challenges. For instance, it is not clear how to adapt the parameters to the changes of network and traffic regimes by algorithms that can run on resource-constrained nodes. A simple and accurate model of the influence of these parameters on the success probability, real-time performance, adaptivity to various conditions as a whole is not available. What is worse, the cost to be paid, in most cases, will turn out to be even higher in a real environment.

Since most appropriate MAC parameters should depend on real operating conditions and specific QoS requirements, the ideal adaptive and real-time approach for CAP should dynamically select appropriate parameters to offer the required QoS support according to various operating conditions.

4.3 Approaches for Contention-Free Period

Based on the standardized IEEE 802.15.4 protocol, timeliness guarantee and adaptive throughput are the most important features that we have to pay attention to. Besides, timeliness guarantee is also appealing to CPS applications. As the requirements of CPS, low data rate, low power consumption and low cost wireless networking becomes more and more significant recently. Therefore, the IEEE 802.15.4 protocol also provides real-time guarantees using the GTS mechanism. This feature is quite attractive for time-sensitive CPS. In fact, when operating in beacon-enabled mode, i.e., beacon frames are transmitted periodically by a central node called PAN coordinator for synchronizing the network, the IEEE 802.15.4 protocol allows the allocation/deallocation of GTSs in a superframe for nodes that require real-time guarantees. Hence, the GTS mechanism provides a minimum service guarantee for the corresponding nodes and enables the prediction of the worst-case performance for each node's application.

However, the GTS mechanism also presents several negative impacts:

(1) It presents some limitations in terms of efficiency and deployment with a large number of nodes;
(2) Since only upto seven GTSs (1 up to 15 time slots per GTS) can be allocated during each superframe, the GTSs can be quickly consumed by a few numbers of nodes, preventing the others from having a guaranteed service;
(3) A node with a low arrival rate that has been allocated a GTS may use it only partially (when the amount of guaranteed bandwidth is higher than its arrival rate). This leads to underutilization of the GTS bandwidth resources.

For a CFP of a length k time slots, the minimum utilization limit is defined as follows in [23]:

$$U_{min}^k = \frac{k-1}{k}, 1 \leq k \leq 15 \tag{4.3}$$

Figure 4.4 presents the minimum utilization limits for different GTS length values, for one node. From Fig. 4.4, it can be understood that the lowest utilizations can be experimented for GTSs with one time slot allocation. This is because the arrival rates of the flows can be low fractions of the indivisible R_{TS} (defined as the guaranteed

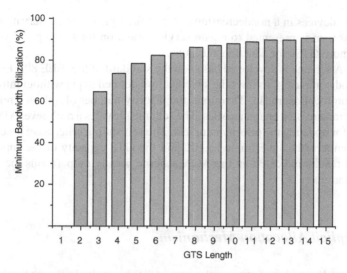

Fig. 4.4 Minimum utilization limits of an explicit allocation. Reprinted from ref. [19]

bandwidth per one-time slot), which triggers the motivation for sharing the time slot with other nodes, if the delay requirements of the flows can still be satisfied. This case is most likely to happen in sensor networks since their arrival rates may be particularly low.

In order to overcome the previously described limitations of the explicit GTS allocation in the IEEE 802.15.4 protocol, a great number of effective approaches have been developed. In the following subsections, we will introduce four popular adaptive and real-time approaches for CFP.

4.3.1 Adaptive GTS Allocation Scheme

Huang et al. [30] proposed an adaptive GTS allocation (AGA) scheme to improve energy efficiency. This protocol is considered to be more superior than explicit GTS allocation mechanism. The AGA mechanism relies on assigning priorities in a dynamic fashion based on recent GTS usage feedbacks with the consideration of low latency and fairness. An ideal GTS allocation scheme has a good estimate of the future GTS usage behaviors of devices. With the estimate, the PAN coordinator allocates GTS resources to needy devices and reclaims the previously allocated but unused GTSs.

To achieve the above goal, the AGA mechanism arranges two phases in the scheme. In the classification phase, devices are assigned priorities in a dynamic fashion based on recent GTS usage feedbacks. Devices that need more attention from the coordinator are given higher priorities. In the GTS scheduling phase, GTSs are given to devices in a nondecreasing order of their priorities. A starvation avoidance mechanism is presented to regain service attention for lower priority devices that need more GTSs for data transmissions.

The AGA scheme is developed based on the standard of the IEEE 802.15.4 MAC protocol and completely follows the specification defined in [1] without introducing any extra protocol overhead. Therefore, the priority number of a device reflects its long-term transmission characteristics. The scheme provides a multilevel AIMD [25] algorithm for updating the priority numbers. The scheduling criteria are based on the priority numbers, the superframe length, and the GTS capacity of the superframe. Numerical results indicate that the AGA scheme greatly outperforms the existing implementations.

4.3.2 Implicit Allocation Mechanism

Based on the basic idea of sharing the same GTS by multiple flows, Koubaa et al. [28] proposed the implicit allocation mechanism. The allocation is based on implicit GTS allocation requests, taking into account the traffic specifications and the delay requirements of the flows. The GTS allocation mechanism is based on the traffic specification of the requesting nodes, their delay requirements, and the available GTS resources [31]. Instead of asking for affixed number of time slots, a node that wants to have a guaranteed service sends its traffic specification and delay requirement to the PAN coordinator. Then, the latter runs an admission control algorithm based on this information and the amount of available GTS resources. The new allocation request will be accepted if there is a schedule that satisfies its requirements and those of all other previously accepted allocation requests; otherwise, the new allocation request is rejected.

The i-Game has the advantage of accepting multiple flows sharing the same GTS, while still meeting their delay requirements. It also improves the utilization of the CFP by reducing the amount of wasted bandwidth of GTSs and maximizes the duration of the CAP, since the CFP length is reduced to a minimum. With the help of network calculus, this GTS mechanism shows how to fairly share the allocation of k time slots in the CFP between N requesting nodes, with respect to their flow specifications. It can be observed from Fig. 4.5 that changing the scheduling policy results in a change of the service curve, even if the guaranteed bandwidth is the same.

4.3.3 Knapsack Algorithm

A knap problem can be formulated to obtain optimal GTS allocation such that a minimum bandwidth requirement is satisfied for the sensor devices. Shrestha et al. [32] have already shown that the Knapsack scheme can achieve better GTS utilization and higher packet delivery ratio than the standard IEEE 802.15.4 scheme does.

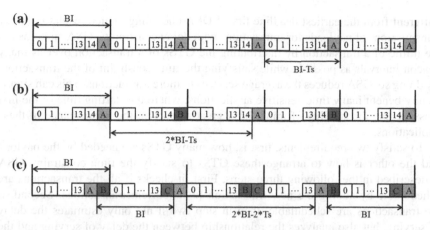

Fig. 4.5 Different implicit GTS allocations. Reprinted from ref. [19]. **a** One time slot allocation used by one node. **b** One time slot allocation used by two nodes under round robin scheduling. **c** Two time slot allocation used by three nodes under round robin scheduling

The main objective of the proposed Knapsack algorithm is to improve the GTS allocation scheme in the IEEE 802.15.4-based MAC when used for a large number of medical and physical sensor devices deployed in a wireless body area sensor network. Shrestha et al. also proposed an optimization model, which takes the priority that is based on the packet generation rate of each device into account. In this allocation model, it assumes that if a device does not send GTS request or misses the beacon frame, it can use slotted CSMA/CA to transmit its data. If the request is unsuccessful, the device waits for the next beacon to send another GTS request. If the packet waiting time exceeds this delay limit, the sensor device simply discards the packet. The coordinator collects all the GTS requests during CAP and solves the knapsack algorithm for GTS allocation before transmitting the beacon frame. It saves the remaining bandwidth that is not allocated for GTS to use in the next super frame. That is the advantage with the minimum bandwidth requirement the sensor devices can still meet their needs.

4.3.4 GTS Scheduling Algorithm

Na et al. [33] proposed the GTS scheduling algorithm (GSA) which differs from the existing algorithms in that it is an online scheduling algorithm and allows transmissions of bursty and periodic messages with time constraints even when the network is overloaded. The evaluation of GSA mechanism is upto 100 % higher than the FCFS-based scheduling algorithm.

GSA mechanism is for beacon mode to meet the delay constraints of time-sensitive transactions in star topology. GSA is proved to be optimal and work conserving.

Different from the earliest deadline first (EDF) scheduling, which results in bursty transmissions of payloads for transactions with delay constraints, GSA smooths out the traffic of a transaction by distributing the GTSs of a transaction over as many beacon intervals as possible while satisfying the time constraint of the transaction. By doing so, GSA reduces the average services to more transactions. This can significantly benefit many time-sensitive applications, where the starting time of the first message and the stability of traffic have great impact on the performance of these applications.

To satisfy two requirements, first is, how many GTSs are needed by the payload and the other is how to arrange these GTSs to satisfy the time constraint, GSA is described in the following three steps. First, it checks if all the transactions are schedulable by adding the new transaction to its current transactions. Second, if the transactions are schedulable, then in step two it not only estimates the delay of serving, but also analyzes the relationship between the delay of serving and the number of GTSs allocated to the delay of serving in each interval. Third, based on this relationship, GSA allocates the minimum number of GTSs to the delay of serving in each beacon interval so that the payload can be maximally spread out. To ensure that all GTSs are maximally utilized and the scheduling of GTSs is optimal, GSA adjusts the allocations of GTSs whenever the payload that needs to be transmitted in a CFP changes. These GTSs are evenly spread out over multiple beacon intervals to ensure a smooth traffic flow between the PAN coordinator and sensor nodes.

Each of these discussed approaches has contributed to improve the performance of GTS allocation mechanism in origianl IEEE 802.15.4. The AGA scheme uses the idea of assigning priorities in a dynamic fashion based on recent GTS usage feedbacks with the consideration of low latency and fairness. The i-Game has the advantage of accepting multiple flows sharing the same GTS, while still meeting their delay requirements. Besides, the Knapsack algorithm, which is based on the solution of the knapsack problem, ensures that the radio bandwidth in the GTS is utilized in an optimal manner. Furthermore, the GSA mechanism smooth out the traffic of a transaction by distributing the GTSs of a transaction over as many beacon intervals as possible while satisfying the time constraint of the transaction. In this way, GSA reduces the average services to more transactions.

Nevertheless, they also have certain drawbacks to some extent. In i-Game and GSA, for example, the information of delay requirements needs to be exchanged with the controller, which incurs signaling overhead. The GSA scheme also has high computational complexity due to the execution of a number of algorithms. In the i-Game approach, since the algorithm starts the GTS allocation from the last time slot in a round-robin manner, it may fail to serve a flow with hard real-time deadline, which needs to be assigned the first GTS in the CFP. Additionally, it requires a control packet for flow specification in the higher layer. The Knapsack algorithm does not provide a detailed priority differentiation mechanism and AGA scheme also has implementation overhead since extra information for devices shall be recorded to allocate GTS resources. Furthermore, energy consumption issue should also be a major concern. All of these above limitations require our future research. In spite of the difficulty of developing an appropriate approach meeting all requirements, we shall do the best to cater specifical needs in different conditions.

4.4 Cross-Period Approaches

In a cross-period approach, the length of CAP or CFP is dynamically adjusted to various operating conditions. Usually, such changes may have significant impact on both CAP and CFP performance of IEEE 802.15.4 protocol. Hence, setting BO and SO has become one of the most important tasks of the PAN coordinator to determine the superframe structure. Koubaa et al. [34] analyzed the impact of BO and SO on the performance of slotted CSMA/CA and showed that higher superframe orders provide better network throughput than lower superframe orders due to their increased immunity against the CCA deference symptom.

Jeon et al. illustrated priority-based delay alleviation algorithm (PECAP) in [35] about how to set BO and SO at the end of the CAP. In this algorithm, the active period is temporally increased to reduce the sleep delay. Nodes having high-priority packets will request the coordinator to execute an extended CAP by sending a priority toning signal. Thus nodes that have high-priority packets can alleviate delay due to the less contentious environment. Figure 4.6 shows the superframe structure when the PECAP algorithm is applied. The key advantage of the PECAP algorithm is that it provides exclusive transmission opportunities to the high-priority packets and transmissions of important data can be ensured with timeliness guarantees.

Another example of cross-period approaches is the AGA scheme [30]. Huang et al. proposed a threshold value T_h, which is dynamically adjusted and depends partly on the BO value, due to the consideration of CAP and CFP traffic load. When the CFP traffic load is light, GTS resources are transferred for contention-based access in CAP to filter unnecessary GTS allocation. Besides, the AGA scheme takes advantage of BO changes flexibly. As the BO increases, there is a higher probability

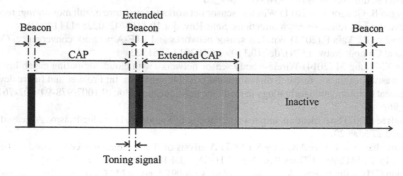

Fig. 4.6 Superframe structure of IEEE 802.15.4 with an extended contention access period. Reprinted from ref. [19]

that many devices have requested GTS service in the superframe. Hence, in such cases, a more strict threshold value is set to prevent the scarce GTS resources from distributing to those devices with extremely low priorities.

4.5 Summary

This chapter pays attention to tackling limitations of IEEE 802.15.4 MAC standard specifications in CAP, CFP, and overall cross-period. A variety of adaptive and real-time protocols have been introduced and discussed. The existing research has greatly improved network performance in terms of real-time and guaranteed communication with adaptivity and reliability. Nevertheless, emerging requirements of CPS demand to improve network performance with possible minimum latency, high energy efficiency, reduced system complexity, and high QoS. Efforts are still needed to develop algorithms and standards to achieve these goals.

References

1. IEEE standard for information technology-local and metropolitan area networks-specific requirements-part 15.4. In: Wireless medium access control (MAC) and physical layer (PHY) specifications for low rate wireless personal area networks (WPANs), September 2006, pp 1–320
2. Shu F, Halgamuge MN, Chen W (2009) Building automation systems using wireless sensor networks: radio characteristics and energy efficient communication protocols. Electron J Struct Eng, Spec Issu: 66–73
3. Yao Z, Sun Y, El-Farra NH (2010) Resource-aware scheduled control of distributed process systems over wireless sensor networks. In: American control conference (ACC), IEEE, Baltimore
4. Marin-Perianu M, Lombriser C, Amft O, Havinga P, Troster G (2008) Distributed activity recognition with fuzzy-enabled wireless sensor networks. In: Distributed computing in sensor systems. doi:10.1007/978-3-540-69170-9_20
5. Aygun B, Gungor VC (2011) Wireless sensor networks for structure health monitoring: recent advances and future research directions. Sens Rev. doi:10.1108/02602281111140038
6. Crosby GV, Vafa F (2013) Wireless sensor networks and LTE-A network convergence. Conf Local Comput Netw (LCN). doi:10.1109/LCN.2013.6761322
7. Xu X, Zhong M (2014) Wireless body sensor networks with cloud computing capability for pervasive healthcare: research directions and possible solutions. In: Frontier and future development of information technology in medicine and education. doi:10.1007/978-94-007-7618-0_96
8. ZigBee (2007) Specification, http://www.zigbee.org/Standards/Downloads.aspx. Accessed by Cited 27 May 2014
9. Ramachandran I, Das AK, Roy S (2007) Analysis of the contention access period of IEEE 802.15.4 MAC. ACM Trans Sens Netw (TOSN), doi:10.1145/1210669.1210673
10. Cano C, Bellalta B, Barcelo J, Sfairopoulou A (2009) A novel MAC protocol for event-based wireless sensor networks: improving the collective QoS. In: Wired/Wireless internet communication. doi:10.1007/978-3-642-02118-3_1

11. Nandi S, Yadav A (2011) Adaptation of MAC layer for QoS in WSN. In: Trends in Network and Communications. doi:10.1007/978-3-642-22543-7_1

12. Lee GW, Lee JH, Lee SJ, Huh EN (2010) An efficient analysis for reliable data transmission in wireless sensor network. In: IEEE Asia-Pacific services computing conference (APSCC). doi:10.1109/APSCC.2010.88

13. Koubaa A, Alves M, Nefzi B, Song YQ (2006) Improving the IEEE 802.15.4 slotted CSMA/CA MAC for time-critical events in wireless sensor networks. In: Proceedings of the 5th international workshop on real-time networks (RTN). Dresden, Germany

14. Zhuang Y, Ma L (2012) An energy-efficient and low-collision IEEE 802.15.4-based MAC for data gathering in wireless sensor networks. Int Conf Comput Sci Serv Syst (CSSS). doi:10.1109/CSSS.2012.315

15. Wu C, Yan H, Huo H (2012) A multi-channel MAC protocol design based on IEEE 802.15.4 standard in industry. In: 10th IEEE international conference on industrial informatics (INDIN). doi:10.1109/INDIN.2012.6300916

16. Wijetunge S, Gunawardana U, Liyanapathirana R (2013) IEEE 802.15.4 based hybrid MAC protocol for hybrid monitoring WSNs. In: IEEE 38th conference on local computer networks (LCN). doi:10.1109/LCN.2013.6761316

17. Yun D, Yoo SE, Kim D, Kim D (2008) OD-MAC: An on-demand MAC protocol for body sensor networks based on IEEE 802.15.4. In: 14th IEEE international conference on embedded and real-time computing systems and applications. doi:10.1109/RTCSA.2008.41

18. Reinhold R, Underberg L, Kays R (2014) Time-critical MAC protocol based on IEEE 802.15.4 IR-UWB optimized for industrial wireless sensor networks. In: 10th IEEE workshop on factory communication systems (WFCS). doi:10.1109/WFCS.2014.6837592

19. Xia F, Hao R, Cao Y, Xue L (2011) A survey of adaptive and real-time protocols based on IEEE 802.15.4. Int J Distrib Sens Netw. doi:10.1155/2011/212737

20. Ko JG, Cho YH, Kim H (2006) Performance evaluation of IEEE 802.15.4 MAC with different backoff ranges in wireless sensor networks. In: 10th IEEE Singapore international conference on communication systems. doi:10.1109/ICCS.2006.301525

21. Chen Z, Lin C, Wen H, Yin H (2007) An analytical model for evaluating IEEE 802.15.4 CSMA/CA protocol in low-rate wireless application. In: 21st International conference on advanced information networking and applications workshops. doi:10.1109/AINAW.2007.77

22. Lee CY, Cho HI, Hwang GU, Doh Y, Park N (2011) Performance modeling and analysis of IEEE 802.15.4 slotted CSMA/CA protocol with ACK mode. AEU—Int J Electron Commun. doi:10.1016/j.aeue.2010.02.007

23. Gao B, He C, Jiang L (2008) Modeling and analysis of IEEE 802.15.4 CSMA/CA with sleep mode enabled. In: 11th IEEE Singapore international conference on communication systems. doi:10.1109/ICCS.2008.4737133

24. Anastasi G, Conti M, Di Francesco M (2011) A comprehensive analysis of the MAC unreliability problem in IEEE 802.15.4 wireless sensor networks. IEEE Trans Ind Inf. doi:10.1109/TII.2010.2085440

25. Rao VP, Marandin D (2006) Adaptive backoff exponent algorithm for Zigbee (IEEE 802.15.4). In: Next generation teletraffic and wired/wireless advanced networking. doi:10.1007/11759355_46

26. Kim TH, Choi S (2006) Priority-based delay mitigation for event-monitoring IEEE 802.15.4 LR-WPANs. IEEE Commun Lett. doi:10.1109/LCOMM.2006.1603388

27. Kim M, Kang CH (2010) Priority-based service-differentiation scheme for IEEE 802.15.4 sensor networks in nonsaturation environments. IEEE Trans Veh Technol. doi:10.1109/TVT.2010.2046757

28. Koubaa A, Alves M, Tovar E, Cunha A (2008) An implicit GTS allocation mechanism in IEEE 802.15.4 for time-sensitive wireless sensor networks: theory and practice. Real-Time Syst. doi:10.1007/s11241-007-9038-x

29. Xia F, Vinel A, Gao R, Wang L, Qiu T (2011) Evaluating IEEE 802.15.4 for cyber-physical systems. EURASIP J Wirel Commun Netw. doi:10.1155/2011/596397

30. Huang YK, Pang AC, Hung HN (2008) An adaptive GTS allocation scheme for IEEE 802.15.4. IEEE Trans Parallel Distrib Syst. doi:10.1109/TPDS.2007.70769
31. Yoo SE, Chong PK, Kim D, Doh Y, Pham ML, Choi E, Huh J (2010) Guaranteeing real-time services for industrial wireless sensor networks with IEEE 802.15.4. IEEE Trans Ind Electron. doi:10.1109/TIE.2010.2040630
32. Shrestha B, Hossain E, Camorlinga S, Krishnamoorthy R, Niyato D (2010) An optimization-based GTS allocation scheme for IEEE 802.15.4 MAC with application to wireless body-area sensor networks. IEEE Int Conf Commun. doi:10.1109/ICC.2010.5502692
33. Na C, Yang Y, Mishra A (2008) An optimal GTS scheduling algorithm for time-sensitive transactions in IEEE 802.15.4 networks. Comput Netw. doi:10.1016/j.comnet.2008.05.012
34. Koubaa A, Alves M, Tovar E (2006) A comprehensive simulation study of slotted CSMA/CA for IEEE 802.15.4 wireless sensor networks. IEEE Int Workshop FactoryCommun Syst. doi:10.1109/WFCS.2006.1704149
35. Jeon J, Lee JW, Kim HS, Kwon WH (2007) PECAP: priority-based delay alleviation algorithm for IEEE 802.15.4 beacon-enabled networks. Wirel Pers Commun. doi:10.1007/s11277-007-9331-y

Chapter 5
An Adaptive MAC Protocol for Medical CPS

Abstract Based on observations gained from the previous chapters, an adaptive MAC protocol called Ada-MAC is presented in this chapter, which is built on top of IEEE 802.15.4 to achieve reliability, real-time transmission, adaptivity, and collision avoidance. The protocol consists of a series of efficient mechanisms such as the time-triggered mechanism, the priority queue mechanism, and the adaptive mini-slot allocation strategy. Ada-MAC not only assigns dynamic GTS but also supports differentiated services for end nodes. Real-time and reliable transmission is guaranteed for nodes with high priority, while data transmission of nodes with low priority is accommodated in unassigned time slots. The performance of Ada-MAC is evaluated via extensive simulations. The results are discussed in detail with a summary at the end of the chapter.

Keywords Healthcare · Sensing · Superframe · Queue management

5.1 Introduction

Ubiquitous and mobile healthcare in the form of Medical Cyber Physical Systems (MCPS) has emerged and attracted much attention from researchers and practitioners. MCPS is an integration of sensing, computation, communications, and medical processes, which can provide reliable and real-time services [1–6]. Context-aware, life-critical, and networked medical devices are used to provide continuous high-quality healthcare for patients within or outside the hospital. To assure safety and effectiveness, numerous challenges are being faced by MCPS. Enhanced viability of MCPS requires developing new standards, protocols, and validation methods.

Generally, MCPS can be classified into two categories [2–5]: (1) Invasive, where in-body sensor nodes are used for monitoring physiological signs; (2) Noninvasive, where on-body sensor nodes are used. These sensor nodes communicate either in star- or cluster-based topologies. On-time communication of life-critical information and limited resources of tiny sensor nodes demand for low latency and high energy efficiency. In order to investigate the performance of IEEE 802.15.4, a number of research efforts have been made in different conditions [7–13]. From these studies,

© The Author(s) 2015
F. Xia and A. Rahim, *MAC Protocols for Cyber-Physical Systems*,
SpringerBriefs in Computer Science, DOI 10.1007/978-3-662-46361-1_5

it has been revealed that IEEE 802.15.4 has the problem of latency and unreliability. To overcome these problems, many ideas and solutions have been proposed so far [14–21]. As an effort in this line, we presented an adaptive MAC protocol called Ada-MAC published in Telecommunication Systems [1]. This protocol implants priority queue and time-triggered mechanism into the IEEE 802.15.4 protocol and supports adaptive GTS allocation to improve utilization of CFP. Details will be given in the following sections.

5.2 The Ada-MAC Protocol

The Ada-MAC protocol is a hybrid MAC protocol, which combines schedule-based on Time-Triggered Protocol (TTP) and the contention-based CSMA/CA mechanism. It enables real-time transmissions and provides collision avoidance by using the GTS policy, and also can adjust the CFP durations adaptively. Meanwhile, the protocol can allocate appropriate numbers of time slots for the particular node that has burst or important data to transmit based on the time-triggered mechanism, while other nodes will transmit their data in the left slots using CSMA/CA mechanism.

5.2.1 Superframe Structure

The Ada-MAC protocol is designed based on the beacon-enabled IEEE 802.15.4 MAC in a star topology network. The superframe structure of the protocol is shown in Fig. 5.1.

The superframe is divided into a fixed number of mini-slots (current implementation is 64; it can be adjusted according to application's requirements) and each

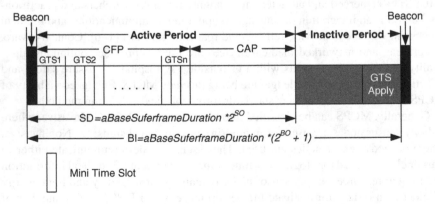

Fig. 5.1 Structure of superframe

mini-slot is capable to accommodate the transmission of one data packet. Beacon frames are broadcasted periodically by coordinator in order to specify new superframe structure. Superframe information includes preallocated mini-slots, duration of CFP, starting interval of CAP, beacon interval, etc. Whenever a beacon frame is received by an end node, it should synchronize itself with coordinator. In time-triggered mechanism, synchronization is a key step to be performed by end nodes.

The superframe can be subdivided into the following three periods: (1) CFP; (2) CAP; (3) Inactive period. In beacon-enabled IEEE 802.15.4 superframe structure, the CAP duration is followed by CFP duration. In Ada-MAC, however, CAP and CFP are swapped and CFP is followed by CAP in order to prioritize data communication of nodes with preassigned GTS.

The CFP contains a number of GTS allocated by the PAN coordinator to the specific nodes for sending real-time data. Each GTS may contain one or more mini-slots and only belongs to one node. The CFP uses the time-triggered mechanism and each node can be triggered at the start of its own GTS and transmits burst and periodic data according to GTS information announced previously in the beacon frame of the current superframe. When its own GTS expires, the node would turn off the transceiver and switch to sleep mode. The GTS assignment for a node is valid only in the current superframe. Consequently, it can optimize the passive GTS deallocation scheme. The transmissions during the CFP can provide reliability and real-time guarantees for the time-critical data. In addition, we remove the seven GTSs per superframe restriction in Ada-MAC protocol. The maximum duration of CFP can be dynamically extended, even to the length of the whole active period.

During the CAP, slotted CSMA/CA mechanism is used for normal data streaming, however, CSMA/CA mechanism with different parameters (*CW*, *NB*, *BE* and *MaxFrameRetries*) is used to transmit burst data. Burst data streaming is differentiated than normal data to avoid conflict. Nodes are acknowledged for burst data transmission to guarantee reliability.

5.2.2 Priority Queue Mechanism

Three types of data communication are defined by Ada-MAC: burst data, periodic data, and normal data. Unpredictable data transmission for emergency information streaming is termed as burst data. Burst data needs to be transferred immediately. On-time and reliable communication is needed in order to accumulate periodic and burst data, however, normal data does not require guaranteed access to shared medium for transmission. Table 5.1 outlines data transmission priority. The priority queue mechanism can allocate different types of data to separate queues and the packets within each queue are maintained in Earliest Deadline First (EDF) order. The priority queue mechanism can reduce the queuing delays of the high priority data.

For three types of data transmission three queues are used, as shown in Fig. 5.2. The queue system classifies the frames on arrival. Classification of frames is based

Table 5.1 Priority of data

Data type	Priority	Requirement
Burst data	Highest	Real-time
Periodic data	High	Real-time
Normal data	Low	Non-real-time

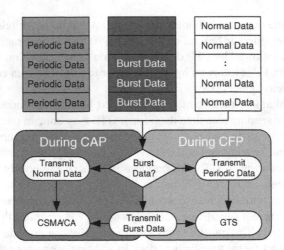

Fig. 5.2 Priority queue management

on frame type identified by upper layer. The classified frames are stored by queue system into corresponding queues. Periodic data, burst data, and normal data are stored in Queue 1, Queue 2, and Queue 3, respectively. Frames with low priority are transmitted in CAP where CSMA/CA is used for channel access. However, in CFP burst data is prioritized and transmitted immediately even both periodic and burst data are waiting for transmission in queues.

5.2.3 Adaptive Mini-Slot Allocation

As described in the previous section, the whole superframe duration is divided into 64 mini-slots. Ada-MAC removes the limitation of fixed number of GTS per superframe. Nodes are assigned GTS based on the data streaming requirements to achieve timely and reliable communication.

At the end of each superframe, PAN coordinator is requested by end nodes for GTS in the next superframe. In this manner, the unused times slots are utilized in the next superframe to achieve dynamic distribution of resources. Before sending the request, the node will check the number of the burst data and periodic data waiting for transmission in the priority queues, respectively, and also the total average Remaining Permissible Delay (RPD) of them. At last, node records the available information, if any, in GTS allocation request. Using the Adaptive Mini-slots Allocation (AMSA) strategy, CFP is scheduled by coordinator once it receives the GTS allocation request from end nodes at the end of each superframe. Below are some important notations and formulas to explain the AMSA mechanism.

Definition 1: The permissible delay for a packet is defined as the time interval (*ms*) between the packet generation time and its deadline.

Definition 2: The remaining permissible delay for a packet is defined as the remaining time (*ms*) before it reaches its deadline.

Table 5.2 outlines the notations that are associated with the time variable of the packet in the queue. Terms containing subscripts Q and i correspond to the ith packet in queue Q, $1 \leq Q \leq 3$.

As defined previously, each packet has a permissible delay when it is generated on application layer. The permissible delay of a packet can be expressed as follows:

$$D^Q_{(permissible,i)} = T^Q_{(deadline,i)} - T^Q_{(gen,i)} \tag{5.1}$$

The remaining permissible delay of packet $D_{(RP,i)}$ at any time before its deadline is calculated as:

$$D^Q_{(RP,i)} = D^Q_{(permissibe,i)} - (T_{cur} - T^Q_{(gen,i)})$$
$$= T^Q_{(deadline,i)} - T_{cur} \tag{5.2}$$

Equation (5.3) is used to calculate average remaining delay of data in queue Q. $AD^Q_{(RP)}$ presents average level of nodes' remaining permissible delay in queue Q. N^Q presents total number of time-critical data in queue Q. $AD^Q_{(RP)}$ is an important parameter to calculate the K^Q in (5.4).

Table 5.2 List of notations

Notation	Description
$D^Q_{(actual,i)}$	Actual delay of packet
$D^Q_{(permissible,i)}$	Permissible delay of packet
$T^Q_{(deadline,i)}$	Deadline of packet
$D^Q_{(RP,i)}$	Remaining permissible delay of packet
T_{cur}	Current time
$T^Q_{(arrive,i)}$	The time when the packet arrives at the destination
$T^Q_{(gen,i)}$	Generation time of packet
$AD^Q_{(RP)}$	Total average remaining permissible delay of data in queue Q

$$AD^Q_{(RP)} = \frac{\sum_{i=1}^{NQ} D^Q_{(RP,i)}}{N^Q} \tag{5.3}$$

In order to get a fair distribution strategy, PAN coordinator allocates the mini-slots to the nodes according to the value of K^Q. The value of K^Q is dynamically adjusted and depends on the number of packets (N^Q) and the average remaining permissible delay of packets in queue Q.

$$K^Q = \frac{N^Q}{AD^Q_{(RP)}} \tag{5.4}$$

The actual delay of packet can be calculated using (5.1). If the actual delay is smaller than permissible delay, the packet is validated; otherwise, the packet is overdue. Even if the packet arrived at the destination, it still will be dropped. It is an essential parameter for computing on-time delivery ratio.

$$D^Q_{(actual,i)} = T^Q_{(arrive,i)} - T^Q_{(gen,i)} \tag{5.5}$$

The AMSA strategy is described by Algorithm 1. GR represents the GTS request sent by end node to PAN coordinator. This request consists of *length*, *MacAddress*, N_b, N_p, RPD_b, and RPD_p. The *length* signifies the number of mini-slots requested. *MacAddress* signifies the MAC address of node. N_b and N_p denote the number of burst data and periodic data, respectively, that a node needs to transmit. RPD_b and RPD_p indicate the average remaining permissible delay of burst data and periodic data, respectively. GL stands for the GTS List scheduled by the PAN coordinator. It contains three parameters: *startslot*, *length*, and *MacAddress*. *startslot* means the starting mini-slots of GTS allocated by the PAN coordinator for the nodes sending requests. A value of 0 means no GTS is allocated to the node. *length* shows the number of mini-slots for the GTS.

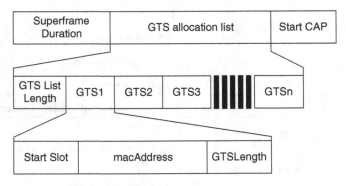

Fig. 5.3 Structure of GTS allocation list in Beacon frame. Reprinted from Ref. [1] with kind permission from Springer Science+Business Media

---

Algorithm 1 Adaptive Mini-slots Allocation Strategy. Reprinted from Ref. [1] with kind permission from Springer Science+Business Media

---

1: **Input:** GR={$length$, $MacAddress$, N_b, N_p, RPD_b, RPD_p}
2: **Output:** GL={$startslot$, $length$, $MacAddress$}
3: $startslot$=1, j=1, m=1, n=1,
4: set $maxslot$ //the max number of mini-slots
5: N=length of GR
6: K_i^b=0, K_i^p=0 (i=0...N-1)
7: **for** i=0,1,2...,N-1 **do**
8:     calculate K_i^b and K_i^p using (4)
9: **end for**
10: **while** n > 0 **do**
11:     $index = N$
12:     **for** i=0,1,2...$N-1$ **do**
13:         **if** K_i^b > 0 and K_i^b > K_{index}^b **then**
14:             $index = i$, $K_i^b = 0$
15:         **end if**
16:         **if** $startslot$ < $maxslot$ and $index \neq 0$ **then**
17:             Assign $length$ mini-slots to the slave node for burst data and since $startslot$, record details in GL[j]
18:             $startslot$= $startslot$+GL[j].$length$
19:             j++
20:         **end if**
21:         $n - -$
22:     **end for**
23: **end while**
24: **while** mn > 0 **do**
25:     $index = N$
26:     **for** i=0,1,2...$N - 1$ **do**
27:         **if** K_i^p > 0 and K_i^p > K_{index}^p **then**
28:             $index = i$, $K_i^p = 0$
29:         **end if**
30:         **if** $startslot$ < $maxslot$ and $index \neq 0$ **then**
31:             Assign $length$ mini-slots to the slave node for periodic data and since $startslot$, record details in GL[j]
32:             $startslot$= $startslot$+GL[j].$length$
33:             j++
34:         **end if**
35:         $m - -$
36:     **end for**
37: **end while**

Coordinator calculates K^Q on reception of GTS request, which is based on the information contained in the request frame: the amount of the real-time data, priority of the data, and the average remaining permissible delay, as expressed in (5.4). This value is used as a threshold for GTS allocation procedure. Burst data is prioritized as compared to periodic data. Similarly, higher value of K^Q is used to privilege data of same priority. In GTS Allocation List, the scheduled information is broadcasted by PAN coordinator. Figure 5.3 presents the GTS Allocation List structure in a beacon frame.

5.3 Simulation Settings

To evaluate the performance of the Ada-MAC, a WBAN scenario is adopted where several in, on, or around the human body sensor nodes collect information from human body and communicate with a central device called PAN coordinator. The sensor nodes can sense physiological signals such as ECG, EEG, blood pressure, temperature, etc. Some of them need to be delivered correctly within a predefined deadline. Burst data is totally unpredictable. It is generated randomly and needs to be transmitted in time. The permissible delay of each data type assumed for simulation is given in Table 5.3. End nodes are categorized into two types: (1) Normal nodes: these nodes are capable to generate burst data and normal data, and (2) Real-Time (RT) nodes: these nodes generate all three types of data. The priority for same data type generated by different nodes remains the same. In order to reduce the complexity of simulation environment and model, several assumptions are made without loss of generality. These assumptions include:

- No hidden nodes in the simulation;
- The coordinator only receives GTS requests and does not transmit; and
- Allocated GTS are considered for uplink data streaming.

The OMNeT++ simulation environment is used to evaluate Ada-MAC, where a star topology with a single PAN coordinator is considered. 20 nodes are uniformly distributed in a circular area of radius 150 cm while PAN coordinator is placed at the center of the circle. In order to provide guaranteed channel access in CAP, priority backoff method is used for burst day in contention. *NB*, *CW*, *BE*, and *MaxFrameRetries* are the important parameters which affect the CSMA/CA mechanism. These values can be dynamically adjusted. The values of these parameters to accommodate burst and periodic data are given in Table 5.4.

Table 5.3 Allowable delay of data

Data type	Allowable delay
Burst data	200 ms
Periodic data	400 ms
Normal data	—

Table 5.4 CSMA/CA parameters in simulations

CSMA/CA parameter	Value for burst data	Value for periodic data
NB	6	3
MinBE	2	3
MaxBE	4	6
MaxFrameRetries	—	2
CW	1	2
ACK request	Yes	No

Table 5.5 Simulation parameters

Parameter	Value
Carrier frequency	2.4 GHz
Network topology	Star topology
Synchronization mode	Beacon-enabled
Transmitter power	1 mW
Carrier sensitivity	−85 dBm
Data rate	250 Kbps
Queue length	10 packets
Traffic type	Exponential
Run time	2000 s
MAC payload size (MSDU size)	50 bytes
Superframe order (SO)	4
Beacon order (BO)	4
Total number of end devices	20 (default)
Number of RT devices (nodes)	14 (default)
The packet generation interval of periodic data	0.3 s (default)
The generation probability of burst data	0.5 % (default)

Reprinted from Ref. [1] with kind permission from Springer Science+Business Media

The values of variables and parameters used in simulations are given in Table 5.5. The performance of Ada-MAC is evaluated in terms of timeliness, reliability, and resource efficiency with different packet generation rate for different types of data streaming. The following performance metrics are considered to fulfill these requirements.

- **Mean/max end-to-end delay**: the average time duration from packet generation at end node to successful reception of the packet at coordinator node. To evaluate the real-time performance, this metric is of great importance.
- **On-time delivery ratio**: this metric reflects the dependability and latency performance of networks. It is computed as the ratio of the number of packets delivered to the MAC layer of destination node correctly before the deadline to the total number of each type of packets generated by all source nodes. $D_{(permissible,i)}$ is an important threshold value. If $D_{(permissible,i)} \geq D_{(actual,i)}$, the packet is validated and the transmission is called on-time delivery.
- **Packet drop ratio (by queue)**: this metric expresses the ratio of the total number of dropped packets by the queue at the source nodes to the total number of each type of packets generated by source nodes. This metric can also reflect the reliability of the network.
- **Packet loss rate**: this metric expresses the ratio of the number of packets lost during the transmission to the total number of each type of packets generated by source nodes.

- **Effective utilization rate of CFP**: this metric is used to measure the effective utilization rate of CFP bandwidth. It indicates the GTS resource efficiency. It is the ratio of the time used for transmitting time-critical packets to the total time duration of CFP.

5.4 Results and Analysis

Like IEEE 802.15.4, Ada-MAC has been evaluated in two different access modes and compared with IEEE 802.15.4. Data traffic is generated using an exponential distribution. Burst data is generated randomly. The probability of burst data denoted by P_{burst} varies from 0.2 to 10 %. The generation interval of periodic data $PGI_{periodic}$ varies from 0.1 to 0.7 s while the generation interval of normal data is fixed to 0.06 s.

5.4.1 Mean/Max End-to-End Delay

The real-time performance is evaluated in three different access modes: Ada-MAC, slotted CSMA/CA, and CFP. The total number of end nodes is 20 as indicated in Table 5.5. The performance is evaluated with respect to different numbers of RT nodes.

Figure 5.4 presents the mean end-to-end delay of time-critical data against number of RT nodes. Figure 5.5 shows the max end-to-end delay for the same configurations.

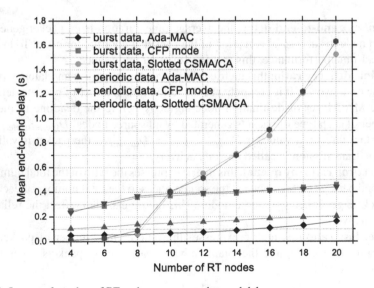

Fig. 5.4 Impact of number of RT nodes on mean end-to-end delay

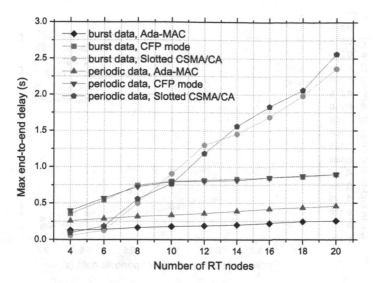

Fig. 5.5 Impact of number of RT nodes on max end-to-end Delay

Significant rise in delay with increasing number of RT nodes is observed for original IEEE 802.15.4 with slotted CSMA/CA mechanism. This significant increase in delay for time-critical data is due to higher contention for channel access with CSMA/CA mechanism, which increases with increasing number of end nodes. On the contrary, in the Ada-MAC protocol, the periodic data can always keep an acceptable latency with the increasing number of RT nodes. This is because in the original IEEE 802.15.4, the buffered packets incur severe contentions and lead to a pretty long delay of real-time data.

In contrast, the priority queue adopted in the Ada-MAC protocol can ensure that the high priority data are privileged to be delivered to their destination. In addition, the Ada-MAC allocates GTS for the burst data and the periodic data dynamically depending on their remaining permissible delay. This method can schedule the transmission order of the time-critical data more reasonably as compared with CSMA/CA mechanism and CFP mode. Furthermore, the burst can also be transmitted in the CAP, which will also decrease the delay significantly.

Mean end-to-end delays of periodic data and burst data with different values of $PGI_{periodic}$ and P_{burst} in the context of Ada-MAC are depicted in Figs. 5.6 and 5.7, respectively. It is observed that under the same $PGI_{periodic}$, the larger P_{burst} leads to the longer average delay. As $PGI_{periodic}$ decreases, the average delay grows gradually. It can be easily explained that the larger P_{burst} or smaller $PGI_{periodic}$ means a higher traffic load which leads to worse competition environment and hence the data will suffer a longer waiting time. Nevertheless, most of the delay of time-critical data maintains within their permissible delay. This is because the Ada-MAC provides a priority queue and an adaptive mini-slot allocation strategy and tries to ensure that the critical data can be delivered to the destination in a bounded time interval.

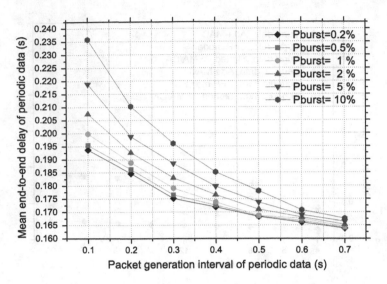

Fig. 5.6 Mean end-to-end delay of periodic data in Ada-MAC

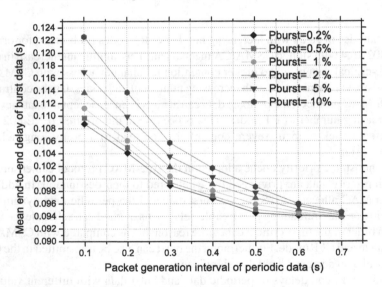

Fig. 5.7 Mean end-to-end delay of burst data in Ada-MAC

5.4.2 On-Time Delivery Ratio

The next performance metric used to evaluate Ada-MAC is On-time Delivery Ratio (ODR). With respect to different numbers of RT nodes, the ODR analysis for time-critical data is presented in Fig. 5.8. It is noticed that increase in number of RT nodes leads to decrease in ODR for critical data in case IEEE 802.15.4 with slotted

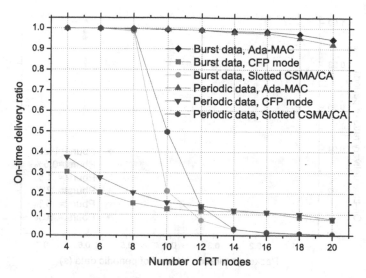

Fig. 5.8 Impact of number of RT nodes on on-time delivery ratio

CSMA/CA is used for shared medium channel access. Increasing number of RT nodes leads to higher medium contention which might possibly cause packet drop. This packet drop increases the delay beyond the permissible range. In case of the CFP mode, the ODR of critical time data is low and declines slowly with the increasing number of RT nodes. The reason can be explained as follows: the capacity of GTS is limited and the data may suffer a long waiting time resulting from the rough GTS allocation strategy before obtaining the GTS. Consequently, less data can reach the destination within the permissible delay. It can be seen that Ada-MAC has an outstanding performance in terms of on-time delivery ratio and can provide highly reliable transmissions for time-critical data including both burst and periodic data.

Figures 5.9 and 5.10 further illustrate the ODR of periodic data and burst data, respectively, in Ada-MAC with different values of P_{burst} and $PGI_{periodic}$. It is clear that the smaller $PGI_{periodic}$ leads to lower ODR. For the same $PGI_{periodic}$, ODR rises slightly with the increasing P_{burst}. Overall, ODR of time-critical data always stays at a high level in all scenarios. One major reason is that the priority queue, the priority backoff mechanism, and the AMSA strategy ensure priority channel access for time-critical data, which avoids collisions.

5.4.3 Packet Drop Rate (by Queue)

Packet drop rate (by queue) for time-critical data with respect to the number of RT nodes is depicted in Fig. 5.11. It is observed from the simulation results that with slotted CSMA/CA, packet drop rate increases significantly when more than

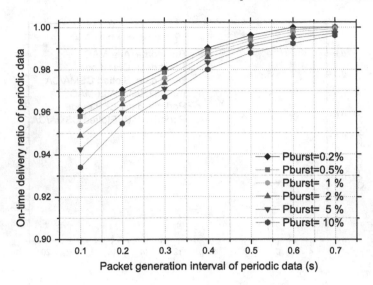

Fig. 5.9   On-time delivery ratio of periodic data in Ada-MAC

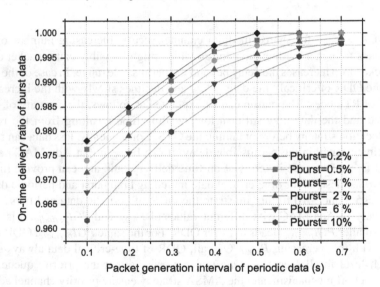

Fig. 5.10   On-time delivery ratio of burst data in Ada-MAC

eight RT nodes try to access the channel. Due to increasing number of RT nodes, intense channel contention leads to longer waiting time in queue, which in turn might cause packet drop. The poor GTS allocation scheme in CFP mode results in the worst performance. Thanks to priority queue management and service differentiation, Ada-MAC is superior to all the other schemes in terms of packet drop rate of time-critical data.

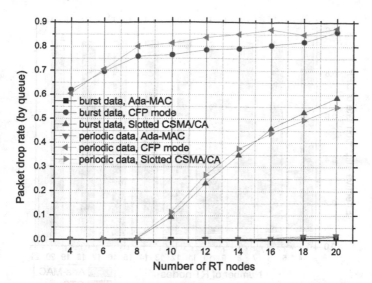

Fig. 5.11 Impact of number of RT nodes on packet drop rate (by queue)

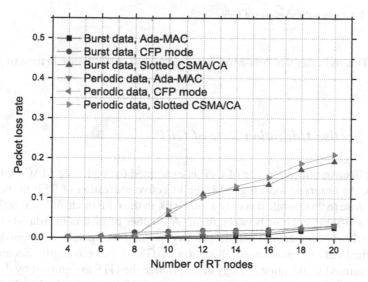

Fig. 5.12 Impact of number of RT nodes on packet loss rate

5.4.4 Packet Loss Rate

Figure 5.12 depicts the packet loss rates with different numbers of RT nodes. All the three schemes maintain a good performance for small numbers of RT nodes. As the RT nodes become dense (i.e., more than 8), the packet loss rate under slotted CSMA/CA begins to incline gradually while Ada-MAC and the CFP mode hardly

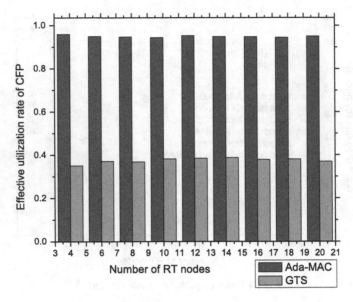

Fig. 5.13 Effective utilization rate of CFP

change. This indicates that Ada-MAC has a very good performance in term of packet loss rate.

5.4.5 Effective Utilization Rate of CFP

At last, effective utilization rate of CFP is examined for both Ada-MAC and IEEE 802.15.4. As observed form Fig. 5.13, the effective utilization of CFP in the Ada-MAC is close to 95 % while it is only about 30 % in the CFP mode of IEEE 802.15.4. There is a striking contrast between them. A number of factors in Ada-MAC contribute to this phenomenon. First, the priority queuing mechanism distinguishes the time-critical data for guaranteed allocation of GTS more efficiently. Second, the adaptive mini-slot allocation strategy can optimize the GTS assignment by dynamically adjusting the CFP and reducing the waste of GTS. As a result, Ada-MAC can yield a much higher utilization rate of CFP.

5.5 Summary

Based on observations gained from the previous chapters, an adaptive MAC scheme for MCPS, called Ada-MAC, has been presented in this chapter. It can guarantee real-time and reliable communication for MCPS over WBAN. Ada-MAC provides different transmission modes for different types of data. It uses a dynamic and adaptive scheme for GTS allocation to nodes with variable bandwidth requirements. Priority queue management is adopted to accommodate burst data. An AMSA policy is used to further improve its adaptability. The performance of Ada-MAC has been evaluated in comparison with original IEEE 802.15.4 MAC protocol in different modes. From simulation results, it is concluded that Ada-MAC significantly outperforms the traditional one, in terms of reliability and real-time guarantees for time-critical data transmissions.

References

1. Xia F, Wang L, Zhang D, He D, Kong X (2014) An adaptive MAC protocol for real-time and reliable communications in medical cyber-physical systems. Telecommun Syst, accepted for publication. doi:10.1007/s11235-014-9895-2
2. Sokolsky O (2011) Medical cyber-physical systems. In: 18th IEEE international conference and workshops on engineering of computer based systems (ECBS). doi:10.1109/ECBS.2011. 40
3. Ullah S, Higgins H, Braem B, Latre B, Blondia C, Moerman I, Saleem S, Rahman Z, Kwak KS (2012) A comprehensive survey of wireless body area networks. J Med Syst 36(3):1065–1094. doi:10.1007/s10916-010-9571-3
4. Lee I, Sokolsky O, Chen S, Hatcliff J, Jee E, Kim B, King A, Mullen-Fortino M, Soojin P, Roederer A, Venkatasubramanian KK (2012) Challenges and research directions in medical cyber-physical systems. Proc IEEE. doi:10.1109/JPROC.2011.2165270
5. Alam MM, Berder O, Menard D, Sentieys O (2012) TAD-MAC: traffic-aware dynamic MAC protocol for wireless body area sensor networks. IEEE J Emerg Sel Top Circuits Syst 2(1):109–119. doi:10.1109/JETCAS.2012.2187243
6. Omeni O, Wong ACW, Burdett AJ, Toumazou C (2008) Energy efficient medium access protocol for wireless medical body area sensor networks. IEEE Trans Biomed Circuits Syst 2(4):251–259. doi:10.1109/TBCAS.2008.2003431
7. Ullah S, Kwak KS (2010) Performance study of low-power MAC protocols for wireless body area networks. In: IEEE 21st international symposium on in personal, indoor and mobile radio communications workshops. doi:10.1109/PIMRCW.2010.5670417
8. Chen F, Wang N, German R, Dressler F (2010) Simulation study of IEEE 802.15.4 LR-WPAN for industrial applications. Wirel Commun Mob Comput 10(5):609–621. doi:10.1002/wcm. 736
9. Gribaudo M, Manini D, Nordio A, Chiasserini C (2011) Transient analysis of IEEE 802.15.4 sensor networks. IEEE Trans Wirel Commun 10(4):1165–1175. doi:10.1109/TWC.2011. 011311.100188 Chicago
10. Li C, Li HB, Kohno R (2009) Performance evaluation of IEEE 802.15.4 for wireless body area network (WBAN). In: IEEE ICC workshops. doi:10.1109/ICCW.2009.5208087
11. Lauwens B, Scheers B, Van de Capelle A (2010) Performance analysis of unslotted CSMA/CA in wireless networks. Telecommun Syst 44(1–2):109–123. doi:10.1007/s11235-009-9220-7
12. Mehta A, Bhatti G, Sahinoglu Z, Viswanathan R, Zhang J (2009) Performance analysis of beacon-enabled IEEE 802.15.4 MAC for emergency response applications. In: International symposium on advanced networks and telecommunication systems (ANTS). doi:10.1109/ ANTS.2009.5409873
13. Noh KC, Lee SY, Shin YS, Lee KW, Ahn JS (2010) Performance evaluation of an adaptive congestion avoidance algorithm for IEEE 802.15.4. In: IEEE 13th international conference computational science and engineering (CSE). doi:10.1109/CSE.2010.12

14. Anastasi G, Conti M, Di Francesco M (2011) A comprehensive analysis of the MAC unrelia-
    bility problem in IEEE 802.15.4 wireless sensor networks. IEEE Trans Ind Inform 7(1):52–65.
    doi:10.1109/TII.2010.2085440
15. Khan BM, Ali FH (2013) Collision free mobility adaptive (CFMA) MAC for wireless sensor
    networks. Telecommun Syst 52(4):2459–2474. doi:10.1007/s11235-011-9566-5
16. Sthapit P, Pyun JY (2013) Medium reservation based sensor MAC protocol for low latency and
    high energy efficiency. Telecommun Syst 52(4):2387–2395. doi:10.1007/s11235-011-9551-z
17. Kim M, Kang CH (2010) Priority-based service-differentiation scheme for IEEE 802.15.4
    sensor networks in nonsaturation environments. IEEE Trans Veh Technol 59(7):3524–3535.
    doi:10.1109/TVT.2010.2046757
18. Kim EJ, Kim M, Youm SK, Choi S, Kang CH (2007) Priority-based service differentiation
    scheme for IEEE 802.15.4 sensor networks. AEU-Int J Electron Commun 61(2):69–81
19. Jeon J, Lee JW, Kim HS, Kwon WH (2007) PECAP: priority-based delay alleviation algorithm
    for IEEE 802.15.4 beacon-enabled networks. Wirel Pers Commun 43(4):1625–1631. doi:10.
    1007/s11277-007-9331-y
20. Ndih EDN, Khaled N, De Micheli G (2009) An analytical model for the contention access period
    of the slotted IEEE 802.15.4 with service differentiation. In: IEEE international conference on
    communications. doi:10.1109/ICC.2009.5198719
21. Koubaa A, Alves M, Tovar E (2006) i-GAME: an implicit GTS allocation mechanism in IEEE
    802.15.4 for time-sensitive wireless sensor networks. In: 18th Euromicro conference on real-
    time systems. doi:10.1109/ECRTS.2006.13

Chapter 6
Conclusion

Abstract We conclude the book in this chapter. Different MAC protocols for CPS to achieve QoS are analyzed in this book for which IEEE 802.15.4 falls in short. In order to overcome the shortcoming of IEEE 802.15.4, a number of adaptive and real-time protocols have been presented and discussed. This research has greatly improved network performance in terms of real-time and guaranteed communication with improved QoS. In spite of that, emerging CPS require to improve network performance with possible minimum latency, high energy efficiency, reduced system complexity, and high QoS. Based on our observation, an adaptive MAC scheme for MCPS, called Ada-MAC, has been proposed. It is concluded from the simulation results that Ada-MAC significantly outperforms in terms of reliability and real-time guaranteed data transmission for time-critical applications. Finally, we point out the open research issues.

Keywords Network performance · Reliability · Packet loss · End-to-end delay · Medium access

6.1 Summary of the Book

This book provides the in-depth literature review of diverse MAC protocols for achieving real-time and reliable communication in the context of CPS. In this book, we introduce CPS with focus on prominent applications and requirements. Before going into details on MAC protocols, we introduce WBAN as one of the most important applications of CPS, with focus on its architecture, design issues, and challenges. Further, we present the classification of MAC protocols based on medium access mechanism followed by a number of MAC protocols to visualize the efforts made to improve the performance of CPS in the context of WBAN.

As IEEE 802.15.4 was not designed for networks that provide guaranteed QoS, the performance of CPS applications usually depends highly on QoS of the underlying networks. This book includes the performance analysis of IEEE 802.15.4 in the context of CPS. The network QoS is characterized by several metrics, including effective data rate, packet loss rate, and end-to-end delay. These metrics are analyzed

© The Author(s) 2015
F. Xia and A. Rahim, *MAC Protocols for Cyber-Physical Systems*,
SpringerBriefs in Computer Science, DOI 10.1007/978-3-662-46361-1_6

with respect to some important and variable protocol parameters. The analysis of simulation results provides some insights for configuring and optimizing the IEEE 802.15.4 MAC protocol for CPS applications. Some interesting mechanisms, from the literature, used to overcome the limitations of IEEE 802.15.4 are presented in this book.

In addition, based on these observations and analysis, an adaptive MAC protocol is proposed for medical CPS which is built on the top of IEEE 802.15.4. The evaluation of this proposed protocol exemplifies how to facilitate real-time and reliable communication in CPS by exploiting IEEE 802.15.4 MAC protocol.

6.2 Open Issues

In the modern era, reliability as well as efficiency are of great interest to humans. The dedicated embedded devices and computer-controlled programs have greatly contributed to boost the performance and efficiency of different applications in our daily life. However, in case of CPS, where stand-alone devices are transformed into network-controlled devices, applications highly depend on high QoS including improved efficiency and reliability. Deployment of CPS into real-time application, e.g., healthcare and monitoring, demand for high reliability, improved efficiency, robustness to unexpected conditions, and adaptability to system failure. In order to accommodate newly added subsystem or modification, CPS also requires scalability, not only on small scale but also for complex applications.

To achieve the highest level of satisfaction for applications' requirements, metrics like timeliness, robustness, security, reliability, predictability, efficiency, and many others can be used to define QoS. The level of satisfaction varies for different applications depending upon the natural and environmental factors. In general, delay, jitter, throughput, and packet loss are the most fundamental characteristics to define the degree of satisfaction in cyber world [1–5]. The performance of cyber-physical applications usually depends highly on QoS of the underlying networks. However, IEEE 802.15.4 does not provide any means of differentiated services to improve QoS for time-critical and delay-sensitive applications of CPS. The existing research has greatly improved network performance in terms of real-time and guaranteed communication with adaptivity and reliability. The proposed protocol Ada-MAC has significantly improved performance in terms of reliability and real-time guaranteed communication. Nevertheless, emerging requirements of CPS demand to improve network performance with possible minimum latency, high energy efficiency, reduced system complexity, and high QoS. Efforts are still needed to develop algorithms and standards to achieve these goals.

Besides, energy efficiency is one the most important goals to be achieved in CPS. Data streaming of critical and noncritical data, collected from physical objects/environment, via wireless channel is an energy consuming process. It has been the focus of researchers to improve the performance of CPS in terms of reliability and energy efficiency at MAC layer. However, other techniques including, e.g., cross-layer approach, antenna design, and radio frequency (RF) communication and propagation models also affect the performance of CPS. Mobility, transparency, interoperability, security, and high QoS are the other main issues to be considered by researchers for improved and high-quality communication in CPS.

References

1. Lee EA (2008) Cyber physical systems: design challenges. In: 11th IEEE international symposium on object oriented real-time distributed computing (ISORC). doi:10.1109/ISORC. 2008.25
2. Derler P, Lee EA, Vincentelli AS (2012) Modeling cyber-physical systems. Proc IEEE 100(1):13–28. doi:10.1109/JPROC.2011.2160929
3. Sha L, Gopalakrishnan S, Liu X, Wang Q (2009) Cyber-physical systems: a new frontier. Mach Learn Cyber Trust 2:3–13. doi:10.1007/978-0-387-88735-7_1
4. Shi J, Wan J, Yan H, Suo H (2011) Survey of cyber-physical systems. Int Conf Wirel Commun Signal Proc (WCSP). doi:10.1109/WCSP.2011.6096958
5. Mahapatro J, Misra S, Mahadevappa M, Islam N (2014) Interference-aware MAC scheduling and admission control for multiple mobile WBANs used in healthcare monitoring. Int J Commun Syst. doi:10.1002/dac.2768

Printed in the United States
By Bookmasters